MCQs in Pharmaceutical Calculations

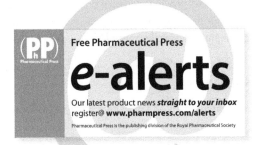

TOMORROW'S PHARMACIST

Welcome to *Tomorrow's Pharmacist* series – helping you with your future career in pharmacy.

Like the journal, book titles under this banner are specifically aimed at pre-registration trainees and pharmacy students, to help them prepare for their future career. These books provide guidance on topics such as the interview and application process for the pre-registration year, the registration examination and future employment in a specific speciality.

The annual journal *Tomorrow's Pharmacist* will contain information and excerpts from the books in this series.

You can find more information on the journal at www.pjonline.com/tp

Titles in the series so far include:

- *The Pre-registration Interview: Preparation for the application process*
- *Registration Exam Questions*
- *MCQs in Pharmaceutical Calculations.*

MCQs in Pharmaceutical Calculations

Ryan F Donnelly

BSc PhD PGCHET MRSC MPSNI

Lecturer in Pharmaceutics
School of Pharmacy
Queen's University Belfast, Belfast, UK

Johanne Barry

BSc DipCommPharm PGCHET MPSNI

Teaching Fellow
School of Pharmacy
Queen's University Belfast, Belfast, UK

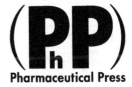

Pharmaceutical Press

Published by the Pharmaceutical Press

66-68 East Smithfield, London E1W 1AW, UK

© Pharmaceutical Press 2009

(**PP**) is a trademark of Pharmaceutical Press

Pharmaceutical Press is the publishing division of the Royal Pharmaceutical Society

First published 2009
Reprinted 2010, 2011, 2012, 2013, 2014, 2015, 2017, 2018, 2021(twice)

Typeset by Photoprint Typesetters, Torquay, Devon
Printed in Great Britain by TJ Books Limited, Padstow, Cornwall

ISBN 978 0 85369 836 4

A catalogue record for this book is available from the British Library

---

Disclaimer

The views expressed in this book are solely those of the author and do not
necessarily reflect the views or policies of the Royal Pharmaceutical Society of
Great Britain.

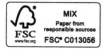

MIX
Paper from
responsible sources
FSC® C013056

Contents

Preface   *vii*
About the authors   *xi*
How to use this book   *xiii*

1 Manipulation of formulae and dilutions   1

Questions   2

Answers   19

2 Dosing   33

Questions   34

Answers   52

3 Pharmacokinetics   65

Questions   66

Answers   87

4 Formulation and dispensing   103

Questions   104

Answers   123

5 Pharmaceutical chemistry   137

Questions   138

Answers   156

6 Practice tests   169

   Practice test 1   169

   Questions   169

   Answers   176

   Practice test 2   182

   Questions   182

   Answers   188

   Practice test 3   193

   Questions   193

   Answers   199

Index   *205*

Preface

The Nuffield Review of 14–19 Learning[1] questioned staff at 16 universities and reported that university admissions tutors and lecturers believe that admitted students are increasingly less capable. There was particular concern about standards in mathematics. Within this report Wilde *et al.* report, as a matter of general opinion, that students reach university with a lower level of numeracy than in the past. In addition, there is a perception among higher education lecturers of a general decline in mathematical fluency, as well as general concerns about basic numeracy skills.[1] It was reported that some lecturers are forced to postpone starting undergraduate courses so that students could be 'brought up to speed'. There was particular concern about numerical competence in those subjects that rely on mathematical knowledge and the ability to apply concepts. This applies to mathematics degrees, of course, but also to engineering, business studies, IT, chemistry, physics and medical sciences, such as pharmacy. Although such concerns may seem a recent phenomenon, those teaching life science undergraduates expressed their growing anxieties that many of their entrants were no longer adequately equipped with many of the basic skills that broadly define a numerate individual[2] as early as 1999.[3]

There are many instances in which pharmacists perform simple calculations (addition, subtraction, multiplication and division) as part of their professional practice. These include working out doses, calculating quantities and concentrations and performing calculations related to extemporaneous dispensing. Many community pharmacy owners and managers also perform calculations related to business management on a regular basis. It is vital, therefore, that pharmacists are able to employ their basic numeracy skills accurately, so as not to compromise patient safety or damage the reputation of the profession. Both The Royal Pharmaceutical Society of Great Britain (RPSGB) Accreditation Document[4] and the 2002 Quality Assurance Agency (QAA) Subject Benchmark Statement for Pharmacy[5] designate the demonstration of ability to perform pharmaceutical calculations accurately as essential for successful completion of the MPharm.

The standards of numeracy of pharmacy students were first called into question in 2000, when a pharmacist and a former pre-registration trainee were cleared of manslaughter charges arising from the death of a baby. Although both the pharmacist and the pre-registration trainee were cleared of the manslaughter charges, they were fined after pleading guilty to a charge of not supplying 'a medicine of the nature or quality demanded' – a Medicines Act 1968 offence.[6] It has been claimed that pharmacy students now reach university with a lower level of numeracy than in the past, and with an almost total reliance on calculators, which has led to an inability to judge the order of number, so that students will accept as correct an answer that is incorrect by a factor of 10, 100 or 1000.[7] Many students also appear to lack confidence in their ability to carry out even simple calculations accurately.[8]

Concern about numeracy standards in pharmacy is such that the RPSGB, the current professional and regulatory body for pharmacists in England, Scotland and Wales, introduced a compulsory calculations section onto their registration examination in 2002. The Pharmaceutical Society of Northern Ireland (PSNI) similarly introduced a calculation element to their registration examination in 2005. Both professional bodies have stipulated that each pre-registration trainee must achieve a score of at least 70% in 20 pharmaceutical calculations to register as a pharmacist. This element of the registration examination must be passed independently of other components of the examination. The PSNI permit their students to use a calculator for this examination but the RPSGB do not. Many UK pharmacy schools have altered their teaching of basic numeracy skills to include additional teaching of numeracy and specific preparation for the calculations section on the registration exam.[8]

It is our view that good basic numeracy skills are essential for competent practice as a pharmacist. We agree with the belief that 'practice makes perfect' in terms of being able to perform calculations accurately and with confidence.[9] The recent success rates in the RPSGB and PSNI registration examinations reflect that there is a high level of competence among those new pharmacists entering the register across the UK. In the summer 2008 pre-registration examination 95.7% (mean score of 90%)[10] of candidates were successful in the calculations section of the RPSGB paper and there was a 100% success rate in the PSNI registration exam.[11]

There are many excellent textbooks now available on pharmaceutical calculations, including *Introduction to Pharmaceutical Calculations* and *Pharmaceutical Calculations Workbook* by Rees, Smith and Smith from the Pharmaceutical Press. This book is not intended to compete with these texts, but to allow the student ample opportunity to practise what they have learnt.

It is intended that, through use of this book, confidence in performing pharmaceutical calculations will be improved and areas of weakness identified and dealt with. This book contains 360 calculations questions, in three different multiple choice formats, covering five important areas in pharmaceutical science and practice. As such, it is likely to be of great benefit to both pharmacy undergraduate students and those preparing for professional registration examinations. Unlike other multiple choice books, answers are accompanied by full working, so as to demonstrate the correct methods of calculation to be employed in each case and to aid understanding.

We hope that you enjoy using this book and that, through its use, your competence and confidence in carrying out pharmaceutical calculations on a regular basis is enhanced.

Ryan F Donnelly and Johanne Barry
Belfast, November 2008

References

1. Wilde S, Wright S, Hayward G, Johnson J, Skerrett R. *Nuffield Review of 14–19 Education*. Nuffield Review Higher Education Focus Groups Preliminary Report, 2006. Available at: www.nuffield14-19review. org.uk/files/documents106-1.pdf (accessed 11 November 2008).

2. Department for Education and Skills. *The Implementation of the National Numeracy Strategy*. The Final Report of the Numeracy Task Force. London: DfES, 1998.

3. Phoenix DA. Numeracy and the life scientist! *Journal of Biological Education* 1999; **34**: 3–4.

4. Dewdney R. *Accreditation of UK Pharmacy Degree Courses*. London: Royal Pharmaceutical Society of Great Britain, 2000.

5 Quality Assurance Agency for Higher Education. *Pharmacy Subject Benchmark Statements*. Gloucester: Quality Assurance Agency for Higher Education, 2002. Available at: www.qaa.ac.uk/ academicinfrastructure/benchmark/honours/pharmacy.asp (accessed 11 November 2008).

6. Anon. Boots Pharmacist and trainee cleared of baby's manslaughter, but fined for dispensing a defective medicine. *Pharmaceutical Journal* 2000; **264**: 390–392.

7. Nathan, A. (2000) 'Poor numeracy of students.' *The Pharmaceutical Journal* 264: 592.

8. Barry JG, Colville JA, Donnelly RF. Attitudes of pharmacy students and community pharmacist to numeracy. *Pharmacy Education* 2007; 7: 123–131.

9. Grandelli-Niemi H, Hupli M, Leino-Kilpi H, Puukka P. Medication calculation skills of nurses in Finland. *Journal of Clinical Nursing* 2003; **12**: 519–528.
10. Anon. 94 per cent pass registration examination. *Pharmaceutical Journal* 2008; **281**: 94.
11. Scott EM. *Pharmaceutical Society of Northern Ireland Annual Report and Accounts 2007/08.* Belfast: The Pharmaceutical Society of Northern Ireland, 2008. Available at: www.psni.org.uk/documents/ 182/PSNI_AnnualReport2008.pdf (accessed 12 November 2008).

About the authors

Ryan F Donnelly obtained a BSc (First Class) in Pharmacy from Queen's University Belfast in 1999 and was awarded the Pharmaceutical Society of Northern Ireland's Gold Medal. Following a year of pre-registration training spent in community pharmacy practice, he registered with the Pharmaceutical Society of Northern Ireland. He then returned to the School of Pharmacy in 2000 to undertake a PhD in Pharmaceutics. He graduated in 2003 and, after a short period of post-doctoral research, was appointed to a lectureship in pharmaceutics in January 2004.

Dr Donnelly's research interests are centered on transdermal and topical drug delivery. Recent work has included the design of novel dosage forms containing photosensitisers for photodynamic therapy (PDT) and photodynamic antimicrobial chemotherapy (PACT), and the use of microneedle arrays to bypass the stratum corneum barrier. In addition, he has interests in mucoadhesion, drug delivery across the nail and the investigation of drug–excipient and excipient–excipient interactions within pharmaceutical systems.

Dr Donnelly is the author of over 150 peer-reviewed publications, including around 50 full papers. He is a member of the editorial advisory boards of *Pharmaceutical Technology Europe* and *Recent Patents in Drug Delivery and Formulation*. He also regularly reviews papers for *Journal of Controlled Release and Pharmaceutical Research*. Dr Donnelly is an Associate Member of the Radiation Biology and PDT Group at the Norwegian Institute for Cancer Research, where he holds the position of Visiting Scientist.

Johanne Barry obtained a BSc in Pharmacy from Queen's University Belfast in 1999. Johanne then completed her pre-registration training with Boots the Chemist in England. After spending 4 years in community practice with Boots in both the Republic of Ireland and Northern Ireland, she returned to Queen's University in 2004 to take up the post of Boots Teacher Practitioner in the School of Pharmacy. Johanne then joined the staff of the

School of Pharmacy in 2006 as a teaching fellow. Johanne also acts as a tutor for NICPLD (Northern Ireland Centre for Pharmacy Learning and Development) and has been involved in pre-registration calculation training for the Pharmaceutical Society of Northern Ireland. She continues to work as a community pharmacist with Boots outside of the university term.

How to use this book

This book is arranged into six chapters. The first five cover important areas of pharmaceutical science and practice where calculations are frequently employed, namely manipulation of formulae and dilutions, dosing, pharmacokinetics, formulation and dispensing, and pharmaceutical chemistry. The questions in each chapter are 'open book' in nature and should be able to be performed without the aid of an electronic calculator. Three formats of question are used throughout this book to reflect the formats used for calculations-based examinations in schools of pharmacy and by pharmacy professional bodies. There are approximately 3 hours of work in each of the first five chapters. It is, therefore, recommended that each chapter is not completed in a single sitting. Answers, showing full working, are provided at the end of each chapter.

The final chapter of the book is set out as three multiple choice calculations tests, each to be completed in 1 hour without the use of a calculator. The style of questions used in this chapter, and the distribution of questions from different aspects of pharmaceutical practice, reflects the calculations sections of pre-registration examinations used by, among others, The Royal Pharmaceutical Society of Great Britain.

This book is accompanied by an additional 100 calculation-based multiple choice questions, arranged into five 1-hour tests, which are available from the Pharmaceutical Press FastTrack website. Importantly, these questions are available in the format of both The Royal Pharmaceutical Society of Great Britain and the Pharmaceutical Society of Northern Ireland registration examinations.

As outlined in the preface, the required pass mark in the calculation section of both the RPSGB and PSNI registration examinations is 70%. This mark must be achieved through the completion of 20 multiple-choice questions. We therefore recommend that this is at least the success level that each user of our book should be aiming to achieve, especially within the practice tests of Chapter 6 and the online exercises. If you find that you are not achieving this level of competence or that you identify that there are particular types of questions with which you are having repeated difficulties, you should seek to improve your understanding of the concepts and techniques involved. We suggest that you do this by referring to some of the other textbooks on calculations that provide more in-depth guidance, e.g. *Introduction to Pharmaceutical Calculations* by Rees *et al.*, also published by the Pharmaceutical Press.

1 Manipulation of formulae and dilutions

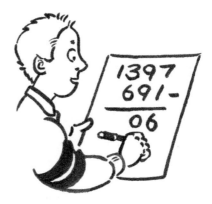

This first chapter of questions is specifically designed to cover a range of numeracy skills. It will give the user further experience in the skills of addition, subtraction, multiplication and division. Competence and confidence in these four skills, along with a heightened understanding of the place of calculations for the modern-day pharmacist, is key to success within the area of pharmaceutical calculations. We suggest for this chapter, as with the other chapters, that students should work in a methodical fashion and clearly record their 'working out' so that they can quickly identify any errors when reference is made to the worked answers. It is also important to show your 'working out' if you are sitting an examination that involves an external examiner, which is applicable to most undergraduate programmes and some registration body examinations. It is important when manipulating any formula to pay particular attention to the units used within the formula and then to compare these with the units within the suggested answers. The concept of dilutions is important and a frequent calculation carried out in practice by pharmacists. If a product is not diluted appropriately it can have fatal consequences for a patient.[1]

After completing the questions in this chapter you should be able to:

- arrange formulae in the most appropriate format for manipulation
- recognise when units need to be changed to be able to identify the correct answer
- demonstrate your ability to calculate a dosage regimen
- perform calculations involving the dilution and mixing of solutions and suspensions.

Reference

1.   Anon (1998). Baby dies after peppermint water prescribed for colic. *Pharmaceutical Journal* **260**: 768.

QUESTIONS

> **Directions for Questions 1–7.** In this section, each question or incomplete statement is followed by five suggested answers. Select the best answer in each case.

1 A liquid medicine is supplied in a concentration of 20 mg/5 mL. A patient requires 40 mg orally three times daily for 5 days, then 20 mg three times daily for 5 days, then 20 mg twice daily for 5 days and then 20 mg once daily for 5 days. Which of the following is the volume of liquid medicine that you will need to dispense?

  A   600 mL
  B   200 mL
  C   300 mL
  D   60 mL
  E   30 mL

2 You are required to make 350 g of a paste that contains 15% w/w zinc oxide. Which of the following is the amount of zinc oxide required?

  A   5.25 g
  B   52.50 g
  C   35.00 g
  D   3.50 g
  E   15.00 g

3 A 1 in 10 000 solution of potassium permanganate contains which of the following concentrations?

  A   50.0 mg potassium permanganate in 500 mL solution
  B   1.0 mg potassium permanganate in 100 mL solution
  C   5.0 mg potassium permanganate in 500 mL solution
  D   1.0 mg potassium permanganate in 1000 mL solution
  E   3.0 mg potassium permanganate in 300 mL solution

4 Which of the following volumes of an adrenaline 1 in 1000 solution would be given by intramuscular injection to a 2-year-old child for treatment of anaphylaxis if the dose were 120 micrograms stat?

  A   12.00 mL
  B   120.00 mL

C   0.12 mL
D   24.0 mL
E   0.24 mL

5   Which of the following amounts of copper sulphate is required to make 400 mL of an aqueous stock solution, such that, when the stock solution is diluted 50 times with water, a final solution of 0.1% w/v copper sulphate is produced?

A   0.2 g
B   20.0 g
C   0.4 g
D   40.0 g
E   50.0 g

6   A child requires a single oral daily dose of 7.0 mg/kg body weight of drug A. The child's weight is 8.0 kg. Which of the following oral daily doses of drug A is received by this child?

A   0.82 mg
B   8.20 mg
C   82.00 mg
D   5.60 mg
E   56.00 mg

7   A patient in one of the residential homes to which you supply medication is going on holiday and needs her prescriptions made up for the 5 days that she will be away. If she usually takes ranitidine 150 mg twice daily and atenolol 50 mg in the morning, which of the following combinations of Zantac syrup (75 mg ranitidine/5 mL) and Tenormin syrup (25 mg atenolol/5 mL) would you supply?

A   50 mL Zantac syrup and 50 mL Tenormin syrup
B   100 mL Zantac syrup and 50 mL Tenormin syrup
C   50 mL Zantac syrup and 100 mL Tenormin syrup
D   150 mL Zantac syrup and 50 mL Tenormin syrup
E   75 mL Zantac syrup and 25 mL Tenormin syrup

Directions for Questions 8–10. For each numbered question, select the one lettered option to which it is most closely related. Within the group of questions, each lettered option may be used once, more than once or not at all.

Questions 8–10 concern the following quantities:

A   100 mL
B   1000 mL
C   4200 mL
D   420 mL
E   4.2 mL

Select, from A to E above, which is appropriate:

8   The volume of an oral liquid medicine, available as 2 mg drug X/5 mL, which is required for a 14-day supply for a patient prescribed a dose of 4 mg drug X three times daily.

9   The volume of alcohol 95% v/v needed to produce 1.90 L of 50% v/v.

10 The volume of concentrated peppermint water required to make 16.8 L of single-strength peppermint water. (Single-strength peppermint water is 1 part concentrate to 39 parts water.)

Directions for Questions 11 and 12. The questions in this section are followed by three responses. ONE or MORE of the responses is (are) correct. Decide which of the responses is (are) correct. Then choose:

Directions summarised:

A	B	C	D	E
1, 2, 3	1, 2 only	2, 3 only	1 only	3 only

11 Which of the following is/are correct?

1   2.0 mL codeine adult linctus (15.0 mg/5.0 mL) is required to make up 100.0 mL paediatric codeine linctus (3.0 mg/5.0 mL)
2   10.0 g calcium carbonate is needed to prepare 1.0 L solution such that 50.0 mL of this solution diluted to 200.0 mL gives a 0.5% w/v solution
3   0.045% w/v is equivalent to 450 micrograms/mL

12 Which of the following is/are correct?

    1   20.0 mg in 5.0 mL equates to a 1 in 250 solution
    2   3.2 g of 5-aminolevulinic acid hydrochloride is required to make 800.0 mL of a 0.4% w/v solution
    3   A 1 in 125 solution equates to 0.8% w/v

Directions for Questions 13–19. In this section, each question or incomplete statement is followed by five suggested answers. Select the best answer in each case.

13 Potassium permanganate solution 1 in 8000 is prepared from a stock of 10 times this strength. How much potassium permanganate will be needed to make sufficient stock solution if a patient uses 200 mL of the diluted solution each day for 20 days?

    A   100 mg
    B   125 mg
    C   250 mg
    D   400 mg
    E   500 mg

14 What volume of phenytoin suspension 30 mg/5 mL is required to be added to a suitable diluent to obtain 150 mL phenytoin suspension 20 mg/5 mL?

    A   75 mL
    B   100 mL
    C   120 mL
    D   125 mL
    E   130 mL

15 Given a 20% w/v solution of chlorhexidine gluconate, what volume is required to make 400 mL of a 2% w/v solution?

    A   40 mL
    B   20 mL
    C   80 mL
    D   2 mL
    E   4 mL

16 Which of the following shows the correct amounts of sodium chloride and anhydrous glucose present in 500 mL of intravenous infusion containing sodium chloride 0.18% w/v and anhydrous glucose 4.00% w/v?

    A Sodium chloride 0.18 g and anhydrous glucose 20.00 g
    B Sodium chloride 0.90 g and anhydrous glucose 20.00 g
    C Sodium chloride 0.90 g and anhydrous glucose 40.00 g
    D Sodium chloride 1.80 g and anhydrous glucose 20.00 g
    E Sodium chloride 1.80 g and anhydrous glucose 40.00 g

17 You are presented with a prescription for allopurinol tablets 100 mg at a dose of 300 mg each day for 14 days, reducing to 200 mg for a further 7 days. How many packs of 28 tablets should you supply?

    A Two
    B Three
    C One
    D Four
    E One and a half

18 An injection solution contains 0.5% w/v of active ingredient. How much of the active ingredient is needed to prepare 500 L of solution?

    A 0.25 kg
    B 0.50 kg
    C 1.00 kg
    D 2.50 kg
    E 5.00 kg

19 A patient taking 10.0 mL Erythroped suspension (250 mg/5 mL) qid will receive how much erythromycin each day?

    A 2.0 g
    B 20.0 g
    C 4.0 g
    D 40.0 g
    E 2.5 g

Directions for Questions 20–22. For each numbered question, select the one lettered option that is most closely related to it. Within the group of questions, each lettered option may be used once, more than once or not at all.

Questions 20–22 concern the following numbers:

A 10
B 15
C 20
D 60
E 25

Select, from A to E above, which is appropriate:

20 The number of days a 150 mL bottle of nitrazepam 2.5 mg/5 mL suspension will last a patient prescribed nitrazepam 5 mg at bedtime for insomnia.

21 The number of tablets required to fulfil the following prescription:

Prednisolone 5 mg e/c tablets
Take 25 mg daily for 4 days, then reduce by 5 mg every 4 days until the course is finished (total course: 20 days)

22 The number of drops per minute required if 720 mL of 5% w/v glucose is to be given intravenously to a patient over a 12-hour period. It is known that 20 drops = 1 mL.

Directions for Questions 23 and 24. The questions in this section are followed by three responses. **ONE** or **MORE** of the responses is (are) correct. Decide which of the responses is (are) correct. Then choose:

Directions summarised:

A	B	C	D	E
1, 2, 3	1, 2 only	2, 3 only	1 only	3 only

23 Which of the following is/are correct?

1 In order to make 250 g of 0.5% w/w salicylic acid in Hydrous Ointment, BP, 1.25 g salicylic acid is required

2 400 mL of a 1 in 2000 solution of proflavine hemisulphate contains 0.02 g of the drug

3   4 × 100 mg spironolactone tablets will be required to make 100 mL of a 25 mg/5 mL spironolactone suspension for a patient who is unable to swallow solids

24   Which of the following is/are correct?

     1   A patient weighing 12.5 kg requires an oral daily dose of trimethoprim 2 mg/kg for 10 days. You would need to supply 25 mL trimethoprim suspension 50 mg/5 mL

     2   560 mL cimetidine suspension 200 mg/5 mL is required to be sent to a nursing home resident to cover a 28-day supply if the resident takes 400 mg twice daily

     3   A patient requires four tablets a day for 56 days; you would supply 224 tablets

Directions for Questions 25–31. In this section, each question or incomplete statement is followed by five suggested answers. Select the best answer in each case.

25   In your pharmacy you have a stock solution of drug F with a concentration of 25% w/v. Drug F is used as a mouthwash at a concentration of 0.25% w/v. You are requested to supply 50 mL of a solution of intermediate strength, such that the patient will dilute this solution 1 in 20 to get the correct concentration immediately before use. Which of the following should be the concentration of the intermediate solution?

     A   5% w/v
     B   10% w/v
     C   2.5% w/v
     D   0.5% w/v
     E   15% w/v

26   You receive a prescription for phenindione tablets 50 mg with the following instructions: '200 mg on day 1, 100 mg on day 2 and then 50 mg daily thereafter'. Mitte: 56 days' supply.
Which of the following is the correct quantity to supply?

     A   60 tablets
     B   84 tablets
     C   56 tablets
     D   120 tablets
     E   90 tablets

27 An ointment contains 1% w/w calamine. Which of the following is the amount of calamine powder that should be added to 200 g of the ointment to produce a 4% w/w calamine ointment?

    A   0.625 g
    B   6.250 g
    C   62.50 g
    D   5.0 g
    E   50.0 g

28 A patient weighing 30 kg requires a single oral daily dose of 9 mg/kg of drug B. This drug is available only as a suspension of 15 mg/5 mL. How much suspension would you supply?

    A   1350 mL
    B   45 mL
    C   50 mL
    D   100 mL
    E   90 mL

29 Which of the following is the volume of a 6% w/v solution that is required to give a single dose of 12 mg?

    A   4.0 mL
    B   2.0 mL
    C   0.2 mL
    D   0.5 mL
    E   1.0 mL

30 Fertiliser residues are sometimes found in drinking water in rural areas. For compound Z, the safe limit for drinking water is 9 ppm. Analytical results for the amount of compound Z in the drinking water of various villages are given below. Which **ONE** of the following villages has drinking water that is safe to drink?

    A   Toome: 24.6 micrograms/mL
    B   Blackhill: 0.3 mg/L
    C   Drumhowan: 0.009% w/v
    D   Magheracloone: 0.041% w/v
    E   Annagassan: 1 in 100 000

31 Which of the following is the concentration of a solution prepared by dissolving 400 mg potassium permanganate in water and making up to a final volume of 4.0 L.

A   4% w/v
B   1% w/v
C   0.4% w/v
D   0.1% w/v
E   0.01% w/v

Directions for Questions 32–34. For each numbered question, select the one lettered option that is most closely related to it. Within the group of questions, each lettered option may be used once, more than once or not at all.

Questions 32, 33 and 34 concern the following quantities:

A   0.8 mL
B   8.0 mL
C   150.0 mL
D   0.15 mL
E   1.5 mL

Select, from A to E above, which is appropriate:

32   The volume of amoxicillin syrup 125 mg/5 mL required by a child prescribed 250 mg amoxicillin orally three times daily for 5 days.

33   The volume of a 5% w/v solution required to give a dose of 40 mg.

34   The volume required to give a 15 mg dose of haloperidol from a 2 mL ampoule containing 10 mg haloperidol/mL.

Directions for Questions 35 and 36. The questions in this section are followed by three responses. **ONE** or **MORE** of the responses is (are) correct. Decide which of the responses is (are) correct. Then choose:

Directions summarised:

A	B	C	D	E
1, 2, 3	1, 2 only	2, 3 only	1 only	3 only

35   Which of the following is/are correct?

  1   40 mL of a 5% v/v ethanol solution contains 0.2 mL ethanol

2 1000 mL of a 3% w/v salicylic acid lotion contains 30 g
salicylic acid

3 200 mL of a 0.02%w/v beclometasone solution contains 0.04 g
beclometasone

36 Which of the following is/are correct?

1 Peptac suspension contains 3.1 mmol sodium/5 mL. A patient
taking Peptac suspension 20 mL three times daily receives
37.2 mmol sodium ions from this medication each day

2 A suitable dose of carbamazepine in epilepsy for a child up to
1 year is 100–200 mg daily in divided doses. An appropriate
dose of Tegretol liquid (100 mg carbamazepine/5 mL) for a
10-month-old baby with epilepsy is 7.5 mL daily in divided
doses

3 A doctor requests 50.00 g of 0.05% w/w salicylic acid cream.
The amount of salicylic acid required to prepare this cream is
2.50 mg

Directions for Questions 37–43. In this section, each question or
incomplete statement is followed by five suggested answers. Select the best
answer in each case.

---

37 You mix together 50 g of 0.5% w/w hydrocortisone cream and 25 g of
2% w/w sulphur cream (the creams are compatible). What is the final
concentration of each of the two drugs?

   A 0.5% w/w hydrocortisone cream and 2.0% w/w sulphur
   B 0.25% w/w hydrocortisone cream and 1.00% w/w sulphur
   C 0.33% w/w hydrocortisone cream and 0.67% w/w sulphur
   D 0.67% w/w hydrocortisone cream and 0.33% w/w sulphur
   E 0.33% w/w hydrocortisone cream and 0.33% w/w sulphur

38 A patient is prescribed a reducing oral dose of prednisolone as follows:

   Day 1: 10 mg
   Day 2: 8 mg
   Day 3: 6 mg
   Day 4: 4 mg
   Day 5: 3 mg

Day 6: 2 mg
Day 7: 1 mg

Prednisolone is supplied as 5 mg and 1 mg tablets. Prednisolone tablets cannot be split. Therefore, the patient needs to take a number of whole tablets. How many of each tablet strength would it be most appropriate to supply?

A   Four 5 mg tablets and fourteen 1 mg tablets
B   Fourteen 5 mg tablets and four 1 mg tablets
C   Five 5 mg tablets and fifteen 1 mg tablets
D   Fifteen 5 mg tablets and five 1 mg tablets
E   One 5 mg tablet and twenty 1 mg tablets

39 A patient weighing 50 kg requires a single oral daily dose of 9 mg/kg of drug Y. This drug is available only as a suspension of 150 mg/5 mL. How much suspension would it be most appropriate to supply to provide a single dose?

A   10 mL
B   5 mL
C   20 mL
D   15 mL
E   25 mL

40 You are requested to supply 35 g of a cream containing 20% w/w methylaminolevulinate for use in a photodynamic therapy clinical trial. You have Cetomacrogol Cream, BP in your hospital pharmacy department and can use this as the cream base. What is the formula for your methylaminolevulinate cream?

A   10 g methylaminolevulinate and 25 g Cetomacrogol Cream, BP
B   30 g methylaminolevulinate and 5 g Cetomacrogol Cream, BP
C   5 g methylaminolevulinate and 30 g Cetomacrogol Cream, BP
D   7 g methylaminolevulinate and 28 g Cetomacrogol Cream, BP
E   28 g methylaminolevulinate and 7 g Cetomacrogol Cream, BP

41 You have in your pharmacy a cream containing 0.5% w/w hydrocortisone. You have been requested to use this cream as a base and to add in sufficient calamine such that the final concentration of calamine in the new cream will be 10.0% w/w. What is the concentration of hydrocortisone in the new cream?

A   0.3% w/w
B   0.45% w/w
C   0.5% w/w
D   0.05% w/w
E   0.045% w/w

42 A stock solution of drug G is available at 10%w/v. You need to dilute this with Syrup, BP in order to supply a patient with a solution containing 5 mg/mL of drug G. Assuming no volume displacement effects, what is your formula for the preparation of 100 mL of the final solution?

    A   10 mL stock solution and 90 mL Syrup, BP
    B   80 mL stock solution and 20 mL Syrup, BP
    C   20 mL stock solution and 80 mL Syrup, BP
    D   95 mL stock solution and 5 mL Syrup, BP
    E   5 mL stock solution and 95 mL Syrup, BP

43 A patient is on a continuous intravenous drip of drug B. He needs to be dosed at a rate of 25 mg/h. The drip is set to administer 10 drops of fluid/h, with 4 drops equalling 1 mL in volume. Which of the following is the concentration of drug B in the intravenous fluid?

    A   1 mg/mL
    B   10 mg/mL
    C   5 mg/mL
    D   2.5 mg/mL
    E   25 mg/mL

Directions for Questions 44–46. For each numbered question, select the one lettered option that is most closely related to it. Within the group of questions, each lettered option may be used once, more than once or not at all.
Questions 44, 45 and 46 concern the following quantities:

    A   0.02 mg
    B   0.20 mg
    C   2.00 mg
    D   1.00 mg
    E   0.10 mg

Select, from A to E above, which is appropriate:

44 The amount of phytomenadione contained in a 0.2 mL ampoule of 10 mg/mL solution.

45 The weight of chlorhexidine contained in 2 mL of a 1 in 10 000 solution.

46 The weight of ethambutol contained in 0.4 mL of 250 micrograms/mL solution.

Directions for Questions 47 and 48. The questions in this section are followed by three responses. ONE or MORE of the responses is (are) correct. Decide which of the responses is (are) correct. Then choose:

Directions summarised:

A	B	C	D	E
1, 2, 3	1, 2 only	2, 3 only	1 only	3 only

47 Which of the following is/are correct?

1 125 g porfimer sodium is needed to produce 200 mL of a stock solution which, when 10 mL is diluted to 5 L, produces a 1 in 8000 solution

2 0.02 mL of a 1 in 10 000 solution will provide a 0.2 mg dose of dexamethasone

3 A patient is prescribed three tablets a day for 56 days; you should supply 168 tablets

48 Drug D is given in total daily doses based on body surface area, with the standard total daily dose being 2.2 mg/m^2. Which of the following is/are correct?

1 A patient with body surface area of 1.80 m^2 should receive a total daily dose of 3.96 mg

2 A patient with body surface area of 2.00 m^2 should receive a total daily dose of 4.40 mg

3 A patient with body surface area of 1.50 m^2 should receive a total daily dose of 3.30 mg

Directions for Questions 49–55. In this section, each question or incomplete statement is followed by five suggested answers. Select the best answer in each case.

49 You are providing prescribing advice to a local surgery. To assist in prescribing inhaled salbutamol cost-effectively you need to compare the cost of the preparations listed. Which one of the following is the **least** expensive for a 200 micrograms dose?

A   Accuhaler 60 doses/200 micrograms per dose (£6.00/ US$11.70)
B   Generic inhaler 200 doses/100 micrograms per dose (£2.00/ US$3.90)
C   Easi-Breathe inhaler 200 doses/100 micrograms per dose (£6.00/US$11.70)
D   Rotacaps 200 micrograms × 112 doses (£5.60/US$10.92)
E   Salbutodiscs 200 micrograms/14 × 8 dose refill (£5.60/ US$10.92)

50 It is recommended that fluoride supplements be taken when the municipal water supply has a fluoride content of < 700 micrograms/L. Test results on fluoride content of drinking water from various towns are listed below. People from which **ONE** of these towns should take fluoride supplements?

A   Tyholland: 0.8 ppm
B   Cremartin: 0.6 micrograms/mL
C   Doohamlet: 0.00013% w/v
D   Carrickmacross: 0.00041% w/v
E   Annadrummond: 1 in 100 000

51 A liquid medicine is supplied in a concentration of 10 mg/5 mL. A patient requires 20 mg orally three times daily for 5 days, then 10 mg three times daily for 5 days, then 10 mg twice daily for 5 days, then 10 mg once daily for 5 days. Which of the following is the correct volume of the liquid medicine that will provide the full treatment course?

A   300 mL
B   200 mL
C   100 mL
D   150 mL
E   250 mL

52 A patient requires an intravenous infusion of 0.9%w/v sodium chloride. In your hospital pharmacy department you have Water for Injections, BP and 4.5%w/v Sodium Chloride Solution, BP. Assuming no volume displacement effects, which of the following volumes of 4.5% w/v Sodium Chloride Solution, BP need to be added aseptically to an expandable PVC infusion bag containing 100 mL Water for Injections, BP to produce the requisite sodium chloride concentration?

  A 25 mL
  B 50 mL
  C 100 mL
  D 125 mL
  E 150 mL

53 A patient needs to use a 1 in 2500 chlorhexidine gluconate solution for wound washing. In your pharmacy you have a stock solution of 20%w/v chlorhexidine gluconate. Using this solution you need to prepare an intermediate solution such that the patient will then dilute this 20-fold to obtain a solution of the requisite concentration. Which of the following is the correct strength of the intermediate solution?

  A 0.5% w/w
  B 0.2% w/w
  C 1.0% w/w
  D 0.4% w/w
  E 0.8% w/w

54 Which of the following is the correct volume of a 5% w/v solution required to supply 150 mg of the active ingredient?

  A 30 mL
  B 20 mL
  C 3 mL
  D 2 mL
  E 5 mL

55 According to an official formula for potassium citrate mixture, 300 mL double-strength chloroform water is required per 1 L mixture. A 2-L bottle of mixture is required. If the double-strength chloroform water is prepared from concentrated chloroform water, which of the following is the correct volume of concentrate required? (Double-strength chloroform water is 2 parts concentrate to 38 parts water.)

A   10 mL
B   20 mL
C   3 mL
D   30 mL
E   15 mL

Directions for Questions 56–58. For each numbered question, select the one lettered option that is most closely related to it. Within the group of questions, each lettered option may be used once, more than once or not at all.
Questions 56–58 concern the following quantities:

A   8.4 mg
B   840 mg
C   8400 mg
D   625 mg
E   6250 mg

Select, from A to E above, which is appropriate:

56   The amount of methylene blue in 3 L of a 2.8 ppm aqueous solution.

57   The amount of fluorescein sodium in 300 mL of a 2.8% w/v aqueous solution.

58   The amount of 5-aminolevulinic acid hydrochloride in 25 g of a 25% w/w cream.

Directions for Questions 59 and 60. The questions in this section are followed by three responses. **ONE** or **MORE** of the responses is (are) correct. Decide which of the responses is (are) correct. Then choose:

Directions summarised:

A	B	C	D	E
1, 2, 3	1, 2 only	2, 3 only	1 only	3 only

59   A patient needs to use a 1 in 10 000 potassium permanganate solution for wound washing. In your pharmacy you have tablets of 400 mg

potassium permanganate. Using (an) intact tablet(s) you need to prepare an intermediate solution such that the patient will then dilute this 10-fold to obtain a solution of the requisite concentration.
Which of the following is/are correct?

1   The intermediate solution has a concentration of 1.0 mg/mL
2   You need to use two tablets to prepare the intermediate solution
3   The volume of the intermediate solution is 500 mL

60   A patient is prescribed 20 g glucose to be given as a glucose 50% w/v injection at a constant rate over a period of 5 hours.
Which of the following is/are correct?

1   The patient will receive 50 mL glucose 50%w/v injection by the end of the 5-hour delivery period
2   After 2 hours, the patient will have received 15 g glucose
3   The amount of glucose in 30 mL of the injection is 15 g

ANSWERS

1 C
Each 5 mL of the liquid medicine contains 20 mg drug. Therefore, there are 4 mg drug in 1 mL. The total volume to dispense can thus be calculated:
40 mg three times daily for 5 days: 10 mL × 3 × 5 = 150 mL
20 mg three times daily for 5 days: 5 mL × 3 × 5 = 75 mL
20 mg twice daily for 5 days: 5 mL × 2 × 5 = 50 mL
20 mg once daily for 5 days: 5 mL × 1 × 5 = 25 mL
150 mL + 75 mL + 50 mL + 25 mL = 300 mL.
Therefore, the correct answer is C.

2 B
If the paste is 15% w/w, then 100 g paste contains 15.0 g zinc oxide. The total amount of zinc oxide can thus be calculated:
350/100 = 3.50
15% × 3.5 = 52.50 g.
Therefore, the correct answer is B.

3 A
If the solution is 1 in 10 000, there is 1.0 g in 10 000 mL solution
In 500 mL, there is (1/10 000) × 500 = 0.05 g = 50.0 mg
In 100 mL, there is (1/10 000) × 100 = 0.01 g = 10.0 mg
In 1000 mL, there is (1/10 000) × 1000 = 0.10 g = 100.0 mg
In 300 mL, there is (1/10 000) × 300 = 0.03 g = 30.0 mg.
By showing that each of the statements B–E is untrue for a 1 in 10 000 solution, we arrive at A as the correct answer.

4 C
A 1 in 1000 solution contains 1.0 g, or 1000 000 micrograms, in 1000 mL. This means that there are 1000 micrograms in 1 mL. The total volume of solution required can thus be calculated:
(1 mL/1000 micrograms) × 120 micrograms = 0.12 mL.
Therefore, 120 micrograms is contained in 0.12 mL. Accordingly, the correct answer is C.

5 B
If we work backwards from the final solution, we have 0.1% w/v, which equates to 0.1 g copper sulphate in 100 mL solution. Multiplying by 50 gives the concentration of the original stock solution, which is, therefore, 5% w/v.

This equates to 5.0 g in 100 mL. As we start with 400 mL stock solution, we need 5.0 g × 4, which is equal to 20.0 g copper sulphate. Accordingly, the correct answer is B, 20.0 g.

6 E
The oral daily dose required = (7.0 mg/kg) × (8.0 kg) = 56.0 mg. Therefore, the correct answer is E.

7 B
Zantac syrup contains 75 mg ranitidine/5 mL. Her ranitidine dose is 150 mg twice daily. Therefore, she requires 20 mL daily. Accordingly, for the 5 days of her holiday, she will need 20 mL × 5 = 100 mL Zantac syrup.
Tenormin syrup contains 25 mg atenolol/5 mL. Her atenolol dose is 50 mg in the morning. Therefore, she requires 10 mL daily. Accordingly, for the 5 days of her holiday, she will need 10 mL × 5 = 50 mL Tenormin syrup.
As a result, you will supply 100 mL Zantac syrup and 50 mL Tenormin syrup. The correct answer is, therefore, B.

8 D
The patient requires 4 mg drug X three times daily, so needs 12 mg/day. If the drug is formulated at 2 mg/5 mL, then 6 × 5 mL doses are required per day. If the patient, therefore, needs 30 mL/day for 14 days, 420 mL are required. Accordingly, the correct answer is D.

9 B
1.90 L of 50% v/v contains 0.95 L alcohol
95% v/v contains 95 mL alcohol in 100 mL. Therefore, the volume of alcohol 95% v/v containing 0.95 L alcohol can be calculated as follows:
(0.95/95) × 100 = 1.00 L or 1000 mL.
Accordingly, the correct answer is B.

10 D
For every 40 mL single-strength peppermint water you have 1 mL concentrate. Therefore in 16.8 L, or 16 800 mL, you have 16 800/40 = 420 mL.
Accordingly, the correct answer is D.

11 E
1   100.0 mL of a 3.0 mg/5.0 mL linctus contains 60.0 mg codeine; 60.0 mg codeine are contained in 20.0 mL of a 15.0 mg/5.0 mL linctus.

2   0.5% w/v calcium carbonate is 0.5 g in 100.0 mL, i.e. 1.0 g in 200.0 mL, which equals 1.0 g in 50.0 mL of the original solution. If there is 1.0 g in 50.0 mL, there are 2.0 g in 100.0 mL and 20.0 g calcium carbonate is needed to prepare 1.0 L of the original solution.

3   0.045% w/v is equal to 0.045 g in 100.0 mL, or 0.00045 g in 1.0 mL. There are 1000 000 micrograms in 1.0 g, therefore multiplying 0.00045 g/mL by 1000 000 gives 450 micrograms/mL.

Accordingly, 3 only is correct, so the correct answer is E.

12 A

1   A 1 in 250 solution contains 1.0 g, or 1000.0 mg in 250.0 mL. Dividing by 50 gives 20.0 mg in 5.0 mL.

2   0.4% w/v is equivalent to 0.4 g in 100.0 mL or 3.2 g in 800.0 mL

3   A 1 in 125 solution contains 1.0 g in 125.0 mL: $(1/125) \times 100 = 0.8\%$ w/v.

All three statements are correct. Therefore, the correct answer is A.

13 E

Of the diluted solution 4000 mL will be used in 20 days. If this solution has been prepared by a 10-fold dilution of the stock solution, the volume of the stock solution required must be 400 mL. As the stock solution is a 1 in 800 solution, there would be 1 g potassium permanganate in 800 mL. In 400 mL there must be 0.5 g or 500 mg potassium permanganate, so the correct answer is E.

14 B

A 20 mg/5 mL suspension contains 600 mg in 150 mL. A 30 mg/5 mL suspension contains 600 mg in 100 mL, which is the volume that must be added to the diluent. This means that the correct answer is B.

15 A

A 2% w/v solution contains 2 g in 100 mL, or 8 g in 400 mL. A 20% w/v solution contains 20 g in 100 mL, or 1 g in 5 mL. Therefore, 8 g are found in 40 mL, which is the volume required to make the diluted solution. Hence, the correct answer is A.

16 B

0.18% w/v is equivalent to 0.18 g sodium chloride in 100.00 mL, or 0.90 g in 500.0 mL

4.00% w/v is equivalent to 4.00 g anhydrous glucose in 100.00 mL, or 20.00 g in 500.0 mL.
The correct answer is B.

17 A
Three tablets per day for 14 days = 42 tablets
Two tablets per day for 7 days = 14 tablets:
14 + 42 = 56.
Therefore, two 28-packs are required, so the answer is A.

18 D
0.5% w/v is equivalent to 0.5 g in 100.0 mL, or 5.0 g in 1000 mL or 1.0 L.
Multiplying by 500 gives the amount of active ingredient in 500.0 L, which is 2500.0 g or 2.50 kg. Therefore, the correct answer is D.

19 A
250.0 mg × 2 × 4 = 2000.0 mg or 2.0 g.
Therefore, the correct answer is A.

20 B
If 5 mg are given at bedtime, this equates to a volume of 10 mL each night. Consequently, a 150 mL bottle will last 15 days. The correct answer is B.

21 D
5(4) + 4(4) + 3(4) + 2(4) + 1(4) = 20 + 16 + 12 + 8 + 4 = 60.
The correct answer is D.

22 C
Administration time = 12 × 60 = 720 min
Total no. of drops (if 20 drops = 1 mL) = 20 × 720 = 14 400
Drops/min = 14 400/720 = 20 drops/min.
The correct answer is C.

23 D
1   250/100 = 2.5:
    2.5 × 0.5 = 1.25 g salicylic acid
2   In a 1 in 2000 solution, there is 1 g in 2000 mL, or 0.2 g in 400 mL
3   We are required to prepare a 25 mg/5 mL suspension. So 25/5 × 100 = 500 mg, which will require 5 × 100 mg tablets.
    Only 1 is true, so the correct answer is D.

24 A
1   2 mg/kg × 12.5 kg = 25 mg daily
     25 mg × 10 days = 250 mg in total
     50 mg/5 mL suspension × 25 mL = 250 mg
2   400 mg twice daily = 800 mg cimetidine per day, so in 28 days 800 ×
     28 = 22 400 mg cimetidine will be required; the suspension contains
     200 mg cimetidine/5 mL, so 22 400 mg is contained in 560 mL
3   This is straightforward multiplication: 4 × 56 = 224.
All three are true, so the correct answer is A.

25 A
Drug F is used as a mouthwash at a concentration of 0.25% w/v. If this has
been prepared from a solution that has been diluted 1 in 20, multiplication
by 20 gives the concentration of the intermediate solution, which is,
therefore, 5% w/v.
The correct answer is A.

26 A
Day 1: 4 tablets/day
Day 2: 2 tablets/day
Days 3–56: 1 tablet/day:
4 + 2 + 54 = 60.
The correct answer is A.

27 B
Use of simple algebra is required to answer this question:
Initial amount of drug = 2 g
Initial amount of cream = 200 g
Added amount of drug = x g
$([2 + x]/[200 + x]) \times 100 = 4\%$ w/w
Expanding the expression out and multiplying across we have:
$200 + 100x = 800 + 4x$
Subtracting 200 from both sides gives:
$100x = 600 + 4x$
$96x = 600$
$x = 6.25$ g.
The correct answer is B.

28 E
The daily dose required = 9 mg/kg × 30 kg = 270 mg

5 mL suspension contains 15 mg
x mL suspension contains 270 mg
An equation of proportionality can be written as:
15 mg:270 mg
5 mL:x mL
Cross-multiplying gives:
1350 mg mL: 15x mg mL
Dividing both sides by 15 mg:
x = 90 mL suspension to be supplied
The correct answer is E.

29 C

The 6% w/v equates to 6 g in 100 mL or 6000 mg in 100 mL. This can also be written as 60 mg/mL.
We need 12 mg, so the volume required = 60 mg/mL per 12 mg = 0.2 mL.
Accordingly, the correct answer is C.

30 B

First, it is important to recognise that 1 part per million (1 ppm) means that there is one part in one million parts, i.e. 1.0 g in 1000 000 mL. This is equivalent to 1000 mg in 1000 000 mL, or 1000 mg in 1000 L, or 1 mg/L. It can also be expressed as 1000 micrograms/L or 1 micrograms/mL. Alternatively, it can be written as 0.0001% w/v or 1 in 1000 000.
Considering each of the villages in turn:

A   Toome: 24.6 micrograms/mL = 24.6 mg/1000 mL = 24.6 g in 1 000 000 mL or 24.6 ppm
      24.6 ppm > 9 ppm, so the water in Toome is not drinkable

B   Blackhill: 0.3 mg/L = 0.3 mg/1000 mL = 0.3 g/1000 000 mL or 0.3 ppm
      0.3 ppm < 9 ppm, so the water in Blackhill is drinkable

C   Drumhowan: 0.009% w/v = 0.009 g/100 mL = 0.09 g/1000 mL = 90.0 g/1000 000 mL or 90 ppm
      90 ppm > 9 ppm, so the water in Drumhowan is not drinkable

D   Magheracloone: 0.041% w/v = 0.041 g/100 mL = 0.41 g/1000 mL = 410.0 g/1000 000 mL or 410 ppm
      410 ppm > 9 ppm, so the water in Magheracloone is not drinkable

E   Annagassan: 1 in 100 000 is the same as 10 in 1000 000 or 10 ppm
      10 ppm > 9 ppm, so the water in Annagassan is not drinkable.

The correct answer is, therefore, B.

31 E
400 mg in 4000 mL is equivalent to 0.4 g in 4000 mL, or 0.1 g in 1000 mL. This equates to 0.01 g in 100 mL or 0.01% w/v. As a result, the correct answer is E.

32 C
Dose = 250 mg = 125 mg × 2
Therefore, 2 × 5 mL = 10 mL is required per dose
Total required = (10 mL per dose) × (three times daily) × (5 days) = 150 mL. Therefore, C is the correct answer.

33 A
5.0% w/v = 5.0 g or 5000.0 mg in 100.0 mL.
5000/40 = 125
100/125 = 0.8.
Therefore, 40 mg are contained in 0.8 mL, so the correct answer is A.

34 E
As there are 10 mg haloperidol/mL, 1.5 mL must contain 15 mg haloperidol. The correct answer is, therefore, E.

35 C
1 A 5% v/v solution contains 5 mL in 100 mL; accordingly, 1 mL is found in 20 mL and 2 mL in 40 mL
2 A 3% w/v solution contains 3 g in 100 mL or 30 g in 1000 mL
3 A 0.02% w/v solution contains 0.02 g in 100 mL or 0.04 g in 200 mL.
As only 2 and 3 are true, C is the correct answer.

36 B
1 Peptac suspension contains 3.1 mmol sodium/5 mL, so 20 mL three times daily = (20/5) × 3.1 × 3 = 12.4 × 3 = 37.2 mmol
2 Tegretol liquid contains 100 mg carbamazepine/5 mL, so 7.5 mL contains 150 mg
   This daily dose is within the therapeutic range for this age
3 A 0.050% w/w cream contains 0.050 g in 100.000 g, or 0.025 g in 50.000 g. This is equivalent to 25.000 mg.
As only 1 and 2 are true, the correct answer is B

37 C
Final weight of cream = 50 g + 25 g = 75 g
From the first cream, hydrocortisone: 0.5% w/w = 0.5 g in 100 g = 0.25 g in 50 g
From the second cream, sulphur: 2% w/w = 2 g in 100 g = 0.5 g in 25 g
For the final cream, we have:
Final concentration: hydrocortisone = 0.25 g in 75 g = 0.33 g in 100 g = 0.33% w/w
Final concentration: sulphur = 0.5 g in 75 g = 0.67 g in 100 g = 0.67% w/w
Accordingly, the correct answer is C.

38 A
Day 1: 10 mg = 2 × 5 mg tablets
Day 2: 8 mg = 1 × 5 mg and 3 × 1 mg
Day 3: 6 mg = 1 × 5 mg and 1 × 1 mg
Day 4: 4 mg = 4 × 1 mg
Day 5: 3 mg = 3 × 1 mg
Day 6: 2 mg = 2 × 1 mg
Day 7: 1 mg = 1 × 1 mg.
Therefore, it would be most appropriate to supply 4 × 5 mg tablets and 14 × 1 mg tablets in total. Accordingly, the correct answer is A.

39 D
Daily dose required = 9 mg/kg × 50 kg = 450 mg
5 mL suspension contains 150 mg
x mL suspension contains 450 mg
An equation of proportionality can be written as:
150 mg: 450 mg
 5 mL: x mL
Therefore, x = (450 mg × 5 mL)/(150 mg) = 15 mL.
Accordingly, the most appropriate quantity of suspension for a single daily dose = 15 mL.
The correct answer is D.

40 D
First calculate the quantity of methylaminolevulinate required:
(35/100) × 20 = 7 g methylaminolevulinate.
The remaining 80% of the cream must be the cream base, so we need 28 g Cetomacrogol Cream, BP.
The correct answer is D.

41 B

In the new cream, we will have 10% w/w calamine. This means that the original 0.5% w/w hydrocortisone cream makes up 90% of the new cream. Therefore, the hydrocortisone cream has been diluted by a factor of 90/100, i.e. 0.90.

The final hydrocortisone concentration is, therefore, $(0.5\%) \times (0.90) = 0.45\%$ w/w.

The correct answer is B.

42 E

The stock solution = 10% w/v = 10 g in 100 mL = 10 000 mg in 100 mL = 100 mg/mL.

The solution supplied to the patient is 5 mg/mL and so a 1 in 20 dilution must be performed; 5 mL of the stock solution should be diluted to 100 mL with 95 mL Syrup, BP. The correct answer is E.

43 B

The drip rate = 10 drops/h and 4 drops = 1 mL. Therefore, 2.5 mL are delivered in 1 h.

The patient requires 25 mg/h, so there must be 25 mg in 2.5 mL or 10 mg in 1 mL.

Accordingly, the correct answer is B: 10 mg/mL.

44 C

There are 10 mg in 1 mL, so there must be 2 mg in 0.2 mL. The correct answer is C.

45 B

There is 1 g or 1000 mg in 10 000 mL of a 1 in 10 000 solution. So there is 1 mg in 10 mL and 0.2 mg in 2 mL. The correct answer is B

46 E

In a 250 micrograms/mL solution there is 0.25 mg/mL or 0.1 mg in 0.4 mL. The correct answer is E.

47 E

1   1:8000 is 0.0125% w/v

    10 mL diluted to 5 L or 5000 mL is a 1 in 500 dilution

    Multiplying 0.0125% w/v by 500 gives 6.25% w/v, the concentration

of the stock solution. A 6.25% w/v solution contains 6.25 g in 100 mL or 12.5 g in 200 mL.
2   1 in 10 000 means 1 g or 1000 mg in 10 000 mL. There is, therefore, 1 mg in 10 mL, or 0.1 mg in 1 mL. Dividing by 50 gives 0.002 mg, so the amount of dexamethasone is 0.02 mL.
3   This is straightforward multiplication: 3 × 56 = 168.
Only 3 is true, so the correct answer is E.

48 A
1   Dose required = (2.20 mg/m²) × (1.80 m²) = 3.96 mg
2   Dose required = (2.20 mg/m²) × (2.00 m²) = 4.44 mg
3   Dose required = (2.20 mg/m²) × (1.50 m²) = 3.30 mg.
All three statements are true, so the correct answer is A.

49 B
     Consider each device in turn:
A   The Accuhaler contains 60 × 200 micrograms doses at a cost of £6.00/US$11.70. Dividing the cost in pounds by 60 gives 10p per dose
B   The generic inhaler contains 200 doses × 100 micrograms doses at a cost of £2.00/US$3.90. This is equivalent to 100 × 200 micrograms doses. Dividing the cost in pounds by 100 gives 2p per dose
C   The Easi-Breathe Inhaler contains 200 × 100 micrograms doses at a cost of £6.00/US$11.70. This is equivalent to 100 × 200 micrograms doses. Dividing the cost in pounds by 100 gives 6p per dose
D   The Rotacaps product comprises 112 doses of 200 micrograms at a cost of £5.60/US$10.92. Dividing the cost in pounds by 112 gives 5p per dose
E   The Salbutodiscs product comprises 14 × 8 (i.e. 112) doses of 200 micrograms at a cost of £5.60/US$10.92. Dividing the cost in pounds by 112 gives 5p per dose.
As the generic inhaler is the least expensive for a 200 micrograms dose, the correct answer is B.

50 B
     Considering each of the towns in turn:
A   Tyholland: 0.8 ppm (0.8 parts per million) = 0.8 g in 1000 000 mL or 800 mg in 1000 000 mL = 0.8 mg in 1000 mL = 800 micrograms in 1000 mL = 800 micrograms/L
     This value is greater than the specification, so supplementation not required

B   Cremartin: 0.6 micrograms/mL = 600 micrograms in 1000 mL = 600 micrograms/L
    This value is less than the specification, so supplementation is recommended

C   Doohamlet: 0.00013% w/v = 0.00013 g in 100 mL = 0.13 mg in 100 mL = 130 micrograms in 100 mL = 1300 micrograms/L
    This value is greater than the specification, so supplementation not required

D   Carrickmacross: 0.00041% w/v = 0.00041 g in 100 mL = 0.41 mg in 100 mL = 410 micrograms in 100 mL = 4100 micrograms/L
    This value is greater than the specification, so supplementation not required

E   Annadrummond: 1 in 100 000 is the same as 1 g in 100 000 mL or 1 g in 100 L. This can also be written as 1000 000 micrograms in 100 L or 10 000 micrograms/L
    This value is greater than the specification, so supplementation not required

The correct answer is, therefore, B.

51 A

• On days 1–5 inclusive, the patient requires 20 mg three times daily, i.e. $(2 \times 5 \text{ mL}) \times$ three times daily $\times 5$ days $= (2 \times 5) \times (3 \times 5) = 150$ mL
• On days 6–10 inclusive, the patient requires 10 mg three times daily, i.e. $(1 \times 5 \text{ mL}) \times$ three times daily $\times 5$ days $= (1 \times 5) \times (3 \times 5) = 75$ mL
• On days 11–15 inclusive, the patient requires 10 mg twice daily, i.e. $(1 \times 5 \text{ mL}) \times$ twice daily $\times 5$ days $= (1 \times 5) \times (2 \times 5) = 50$ mL
• On days 16–20 inclusive, the patient requires 10 mg once daily, i.e. $(1 \times 5 \text{ mL}) \times$ once daily $\times 5$ days $= (1 \times 5) \times (1 \times 5) = 25$ mL

The total volume required $= 150 + 75 + 50 + 25 = 300$ mL. Accordingly, the correct answer is A.

52 A

Use of simple algebra is required to answer this question. If we call the volume of 4.5% w/v Sodium Chloride Solution, BP added y, and remember that the amount of sodium chloride in y mL of a 4.5% sodium chloride solution is $0.045y$, then we have:
$(0.045y/[100 + y]) \times 100 = 0.9$.
Multiplying out we have:
$4.5y/(100 + y) = 0.9$.

This can be rearranged to:
$4.5y = 90 + 0.9y$.
Subtracting $0.9y$ from both sides gives:
$3.6y = 90$.
$y = 25$ mL.
The correct answer is, therefore, A.

53 E

Final solution = 1 in 2500
Intermediate solution = (final concn) $\times$ (dilution factor) = (1 in 2500) $\times$ (20)
= 1 in 125
1 in 125 = 1 g in 125 mL = 0.8 g in 100 mL = 0.8% w/v.
The correct answer is E.

54 C

For a solution of 5% w/v, the concentration can also be expressed as
5 g/100 mL = 5000 mg/100 mL = 50 mg/mL. We need 150 mg, so the correct
volume is 3 mL. Accordingly, the correct answer is C.

55 D

For 2 L mixture we need 600 mL double-strength chloroform water. Double-strength chloroform water is 2 parts concentrate to 38 mL water. We can
thus calculate the volume of the concentrate required:
(600 mL/40 parts) $\times$ 2 parts = 30 mL.
Accordingly, the correct answer is D.

56 A

2.8 ppm = 2.8 g in 1000 000 mL, or 2800 mg in 1000 000 mL or 2.8 mg
in 1 L. In 3 L, there must be 8.4 mg.
The correct answer is A.

57 C

2.8% w/v = 2.8 g in 100 mL, or 2800 mg in 100 mL. There must be 8400 mg
in 300 mL.
The correct answer is C.

58 E

25% w/w = 25 g in 100 g, or 6.25 g in 25 g. This can also be expressed as
6250 mg.
The correct answer is E.

59 B

The final solution for use by the patient = 1 in 10 000

Intermediate solution = (final concn) × (dilution factor) = (1 in 10 000) × (10) = 1 in 1000

1 in 1000 = 1 g in 1000 mL = 0.1 g in 100 mL = 100 mg in 100 mL = 1 mg/mL.

Use of a single 400 mg tablet to produce a final solution of 1 mg/mL means that the final volume is 400 mL. Use of two 400 mg tablets to produce a final solution of 1 mg/mL means that the final volume is 800 mL.

Accordingly, 1 and 2 are true and 3 is false, so the correct answer is B.

60 E

1   The injection is formulated at 50% w/v, so 100 mL of the injection contains 50 g glucose; 20 g glucose can be found in 40 mL of the injection.

2   As the injection is administered at a constant rate, this is a case of simple proportionality. If 20 g glucose is delivered in 5 hours, then 4 g must be delivered every hour. As a result, 12 g will have been delivered after 3 hours.

3   The injection is 50% w/v, so 30 mL contains 15 g.

The only true statement is 3, so the correct answer is E.

2 Dosing

This chapter gives the reader an opportunity to practise questions that focus on dosing. This type of calculation is performed daily by most pharmacists with varying levels of difficulty and we have aimed to reflect this. The types of questions in this chapter often require referral to other reference sources, e.g. the *British National Formulary*, and we suggest that each student ensure that he or she is proficient in using reference texts because this can save vital time in an examination environment. However, recognising that different texts can be used in practice, we have aimed to include as much information as necessary for each question within our text. A wide range of dosage regimens are used for drugs, e.g. once daily, hourly and weekly. This range of regimens must be observed closely when performing calculations because this can help eliminate some multiple choice options at the start of answering a question. A dose of a drug can depend upon the age, weight and surface area of a patient, so all of these have been included in our questions. It is vital that all pharmacy students and pharmacists can calculate doses accurately because it is a key responsibility of the pharmacist to ensure that medicines are administered to patients at a safe therapeutic level. If a drug is not given at the correct dose, it can have no effect for a patient, if too little is given, or could even be fatal if too much is given.

After completing the questions in this chapter you should be able to:

- solve questions that involve complicated dosage regimens
- calculate the correct amount of medicine required to complete a dosage schedule
- calculate a dose of a drug according to the body surface area (BSA) of a patient
- ascertain for how long particular infusions should be administered.

QUESTIONS

Directions for Questions 1–42. Each of the questions or incomplete statements in this section is followed by five suggested answers. Select the best answer in each case.

1   Mrs A is currently taking Mucogel suspension at a daily dose of 10 mL after her three meals and at bedtime. How much magnesium hydroxide will Mrs A have taken after 5 days of compliant use of Mucogel? (Mucogel contains magnesium hydroxide 195 mg and dried aluminium hydroxide 220 mg/5 mL.)

    A   7.8 mg
    B   780 mg
    C   3900 mg
    D   5.85 g
    E   7.8 g

2   A 10-year-old boy (weighing 30 kg) has been prescribed Rimactane 150 mg capsules (rifampicin) for the management of brucellosis at a dose of 10 mg/kg twice daily for 4 weeks. How many of these capsules should be dispensed for this patient to cover the 4 weeks?

    A   108 capsules
    B   110 capsules
    C   112 capsules
    D   114 capsules
    E   116 capsules

3   Mr B has been started on Cellcept suspension (mycophenolate mofetil 1 g/5 mL when reconstituted with water) after a heart transplantation. He is taking the medicine at a dose of 1.5 g twice daily. How many complete days of compliant therapy will each 175 mL bottle of reconstituted Cellcept suspension provide him?

    A   11 days
    B   12 days
    C   17 days
    D   23 days
    E   58 days

4 The suggested initial dose of haloperidol for schizophrenia in elderly people is half the adult dose, which is 1.5–3.0 mg two to three times daily. A local GP has decided to prescribe haloperidol for an elderly man following this guidance for 3 days initially. Which of the following is NOT an appropriate dose for the GP to include on an otherwise legally written prescription?

   A Three haloperidol 500 micrograms capsules three times daily × 3 days
   B Two haloperidol 500 micrograms capsules three times daily × 3 days
   C Six haloperidol 500 micrograms capsules three times daily × 3 days
   D 0.5 mL haloperidol 2 mg/mL twice daily × 3 days
   E One haloperidol 1.5 mg tablet three times daily × 3 days

5 Arnold, a 5-year-old boy (weight 18 kg) with epilepsy, currently takes Epanutin suspension (phenytoin 30 mg/5 mL) at a dose of 5 mg/kg twice daily. How many millilitres of Epanutin suspension will Arnold take during the month of October? You can assume that he is fully compliant and no spillages or medication loss occurs during the month of October.

   A 155 mL
   B 450 mL
   C 465 mL
   D 900 mL
   E 930 mL

6 A patient weighing 70 kg is prescribed drug C to be given intravenously at a dose of 4 mg/kg per h. Drug C is available as a 10 mg/2 mL intravenous solution. Which of the following is a suitable flow rate for administering drug C to this patient?

   A 1 mL/min
   B 2 mL/min
   C 14 mL/h
   D 28 mL/h
   E 56 mL/h

7 A 7-year-old girl has been discharged from hospital on Fucidin suspension (fusidic acid 250 mg/5 mL) for a staphylococcal infection. The girl has to take 500 mg fusidic acid three times a day for 10 days. How much fusidic acid will she have taken after this 10 days of treatment?

> A 0.015 kg
> B 1.5 g
> C 150 mg
> D 1500 mg
> E 150 000 micrograms

8 Drug D has been prescribed for a 5-month-old baby with a body surface area of 0.4 m². Drug D should be given as a daily dose of 200 micrograms/m² in two divided doses. Drug D is available as an oral liquid with a concentration of 0.1 mg/mL. Which of the following is an appropriate single dose for this baby?

> A 0.4 mL
> B 0.8 mL
> C 4 mL
> D 8 mL
> E 80 mL

9 Emma, a 10-kg 1-year-old girl, is to be administered drug M as an intravenous (IV) infusion 2 hours before surgery at a dose of 7.5 mg/kg. Drug M is available as a 5 mg/mL intravenous infusion and should be administered at a rate of 5 mL/min. How long should Emma's IV infusion last?

> A 1.5 min
> B 3 min
> C 15 min
> D 150 s
> E 300 s

10 Vancomycin hydrochloride is to be administered to a 2-year-old patient weighing 30 lb for the management of antibiotic-associated colitis. The suggested dose to be prescribed is 5 mg/kg four times daily for 7 days. Over the total 7 days how much vancomycin hydrochloride will the patient have been given? (1 lb = 0.45 kg)

> A 189 000 micrograms
> B 18 900 mg
> C 189 mg
> D 1.89 g
> E 0.0189 kg

11 A ward registrar requires an IV infusion of 3 L physiological (normal) saline to be administered over a 2½-hour period. The IV giving set being

used has a flow rate of 10 drops/mL. Which of the following is a suitable drop rate?

A 20 drops/min
B 25 drops/min
C 200 drops/min
D 200 drops/h
E 250 drops/min

12 A patient is to be administered 300 mg fosphenytoin sodium by intravenous infusion. This drug is available as a 10 mL vial of fosphenytoin sodium at a concentration of 75 mg/mL (Pro-Epanutin), which is to be diluted to 25 mg/mL strength using glucose 5% before it can be administered to a patient. How much fosphenytoin sodium and 5% glucose need to be used to administer the correct dose to this patient?

A 4 mL Pro-Epanutin made up to 12 mL with 5% glucose
B 4 mL Pro-Epanutin and 12 mL 5% glucose
C 10 mL Pro-Epanutin made up to 12 mL with 5% glucose
D 4 mL Pro-Epanutin and 4 mL 5% glucose
E 1 mL Pro-Epanutin made up to 4 mL with 5% glucose

13 A patient is to be administered 75 mg meptazinol hydrochloride intramuscularly every 4 hours when required for severe pain. The nursing staff who will administer this opioid analgesic are using U100 (100 units) insulin 1 mL syringes with needles. How many units should be administered to this patient each time of administration, given that meptazinol is manufactured as 1 mL ampoules of strength 100 mg/mL (as hydrochloride)?

A 7.5 units
B 75 units
C 50 units
D 5 units
E 150 units

14 Fred weighs 75 kg and requires drug G at a dose of 4 mg/kg per day in three divided doses. Drug G is available as 20 mg capsules. What is the total daily amount of drug G required by Fred, and how many capsules should he take for each dose?

A 300 mg and 15 capsules
B 300 mg and 5 capsules

    C   100 mg and 5 capsules
    D   100 mg and 2 capsules
    E   900 mg and 15 capsules

15 The recommended dosage for drug H is 3–5 mg/kg per day in four divided doses for children between the ages of 1 and 5 years. Which of the following is a suitable dosage regimen for drug H when being administered to an 18-month-old patient weighing 18 kg?

    A   10 mg four times daily
    B   10 mg twice daily
    C   15 mg four times daily
    D   25 mg four times daily
    E   54 mg four times daily

16 A patient weighs 14 kg and requires drug A at a dose of 5 mg/kg per day. What is the total daily dose for this patient?

    A   70 000 micrograms
    B   70 000 mg
    C   0.007 g
    D   70 g
    E   0.007 kg

17 Breda is 9 years of age and weighs 27 kg. She has been prescribed a suspension of drug C of strength 40 mg/5 mL at a dose of 4 mg/kg daily in three divided doses. How much suspension should Breda's mum give her for each dose?

    A   1.5 mL
    B   4.5 mL
    C   5 mL
    D   6.75 mL
    E   13.5 mL

18 A patient weighing 80 kg requires an oral daily dose of 12 mg/kg of drug D for 14 days. Drug D is available only as a suspension of 30 mg/2 mL. How much suspension will this person use during this course of treatment? (You can assume that the patient is fully compliant and no spillage or loss in any other way occurs.)

    A   32 mL
    B   64 mL
    C   160 mL

D   448 mL
E   896 mL

19 How much of a 4 mg/mL suspension would you supply to a patient who required 12 mg four times daily for 30 days? (You can assume that no overage is supplied.)

A   0.036 L
B   0.6 L
C   90 mL
D   360 mL
E   480 mL

20 A junior house officer (JHO) asks for your advice about setting up an intravenous infusion of dopexamine hydrochloride for a male patient, weighing 80 kg, on the cardiac ward. The JHO wishes to administer the drug at a dose of 500 ng/kg per min. The drug is formulated as a strong 10 mg/mL sterile solution, but needs to be diluted to a concentration of 400 micrograms/mL with 5% glucose before intravenous administration can occur. Which of the following is an appropriate administration flow rate for you to advise the JHO?

A   0.1 mL/min
B   1.25 mL/min
C   4 mL/min
D   8 mL/min
E   0.1 L/min

21 Drug E is available as a 5%w/v solution. Fiona, who weighs 6.25 kg, is to be given drug E at a dose of 6 mg/kg twice daily for 5 days. What volume of this solution of drug E should Fiona be given daily?

A   0.15 mL
B   0.75 mL
C   1.5 mL
D   3.75 mL
E   7.5 mL

22 Niferex elixir (polysaccharide–iron complex) is to be administered to a 10-day-old baby boy at a dose of 1 drop (approximately 500 micrograms iron) per 450 g body weight three times a day. The baby boy weighs 2.7 kg, so which of the following is a suitable dose of Niferex elixir?

> **A** 1 drop three times daily
> **B** 3 drops three times daily
> **C** 6 drops daily
> **D** 6 drops twice daily
> **E** 6 drops three times daily

23 George has been prescribed Solaraze gel (diclofenac sodium 3% in a sodium hyaluronate basis) for the management of actinic keratosis. He has to apply the gel twice daily for 60 days using 8 g of the gel daily. Over the course of the 60 days how much diclofenac sodium will he have applied to his skin?

> **A** 14.4 g
> **B** 28.8 g
> **C** 57.6 g
> **D** 480 g
> **E** 960 g

24 A woman weighing 70 kg has been prescribed danaparoid sodium for thromboembolic disease following the standard directions for patients with a history of heparin-induced thrombocytopenia. This standard dose is 2500 units (1250 units if body weight < 55 kg, 3750 units if > 90 kg) by IV injection followed by an IV infusion of 400 units/h for 2 h, then 300 units/h for 2 h, then 200 units/h for 5 days. Danaparoid sodium is available as a 1250 units/mL injection distributed in 0.6 mL ampoules. What volume of drug will be administered to this woman over this complete course of therapy?

> **A** 13.392 mL
> **B** 21.32 mL
> **C** 22.32 mL
> **D** 23.32 mL
> **E** 37.2 mL

25 You are presented with a prescription for ibuprofen for a 10-year-old girl. She has been prescribed ibuprofen at a dose of 300 mg three times a day after food for 3 days. The doctor requests that she is dispensed this drug as Brufen granules, which are packaged by the manufacturer in sachets, each containing 600 mg ibuprofen. How much sodium will this girl consume through compliant use of this medicine for 3 days, given that each sachet contains approximately 9 mmol sodium?

> **A** Approximately 13.5 mmol
> **B** Approximately 27 mmol

C Approximately 40.5 mmol
D Approximately 67.5 mmol
E Approximately 81 mmol

26 A woman has been prescribed Pamergan-P100 (pethidine hydrochloride 50 mg and promethazine hydrochloride 25 mg/mL) for obstetric analgesia. Pamergan-P100 is manufactured as 2 mL ampoules and the consultant has recommended a dose of 2 mL every 4–6 hours as necessary. In total the woman is given five doses. How much pethidine hydrochloride will she have been administered in total?

A 500 mg
B 0.25 g
C 5 g
D 0.05 g
E 25 mg

27 A 76-year-old female patient, Mrs Chambers, suffering from dementia has been prescribed memantine hydrochloride. Her consultant has recommended that her GP initially prescribes the drug at a dose of half a 10 mg tablet each morning for a week and then increase the dose by 5 mg/week to a maximum dose of 10 mg twice daily, with daily doses over 5 mg given in two divided doses. While dispensing a prescription for Ebixa (memantine hydrochloride 10 mg) tablets for Mrs Chambers on day 17 of her treatment, her daughter advises you that her mother is having difficulty swallowing the tablets but has been compliant to date. You decide to contact the prescribing GP and you discuss with her about changing the formulation to drops. What total daily dose is Mrs Chambers receiving on day 17 of treatment and what dose should you advise the GP to prescribe for the drop formulation for the maximum daily dose? (Ebixa oral drops: memantine hydrochloride 10 mg/g [5 mg = 10 drops of memantine hydrochloride oral drops].)

A 10 mg on day 17 and 20 drops morning and 10 drops at night
B 15 mg on day 17 and 20 drops morning and 10 drops at night
C 15 mg on day 17 and 10 drops twice daily
D 15 mg on day 17 and 20 drops twice daily
E 15 mg on day 17 and 40 drops morning

28 A patient is to be administered 3 L 5% glucose over 4 h. The giving set that will be used for this administration delivers 2 drops/mL. Which of the following is a suitable drop rate for this administration?

A   62.5 drops/min
B   25 drops/min
C   12.5 drops/min
D   6.25 drops/min
E   1.5 drops/min

29 A patient is to be administered lidocaine hydrochloride as an infusion after an initial bolus injection. He is to receive the infusion initially at a dose of 4 mg/min for 30 min, then at a dose of 2 mg/min for 2 h, and then 1 mg/min for another 10 h. During this infusion the patient will have received how much lidocaine hydrochloride?

A   250 mg
B   300 mg
C   370 mg
D   840 mg
E   960 mg

30 A hospitalised male patient weighs 64 kg and requires an infusion of dopamine hydrochloride. This drug is to be initially given at a dose of 5 micrograms/kg per min. The hospital pharmacy currently can supply this drug to the ward only in 250 mL containers of dopamine hydrochloride 1.6 mg/mL in glucose 5%. Which of the following is an appropriate flow rate for the infusion?

A   0.2 mL/h
B   0.2 L/h
C   2 mL/h
D   5.12 mL/h
E   12 mL/h

31 While in cardiac arrest a patient is administered a 10 mL dose adrenaline (as acid tartrate) 1 in 10 000. What amount of adrenaline (as acid tartrate) has this patient been given?

A   0.0001 kg
B   0.1 g
C   1 mg
D   10 mg
E   10 000 micrograms

32 A patient is being given an infusion of 0.9% sodium chloride. Which of the following is the concentration of the infusion that she is receiving? (Atomic number of sodium: 23; atomic number of chlorine: 35.5.)

A Approximately 100 mmol/L
B Approximately 134 mmol/L
C Approximately 154 mmol/L
D Approximately 160 mmol/L
E Approximately 271 mmol/L

33 A 2-month-old baby needs to be given fluconazole for a candidal infection. The standard dose of fluconazole for this indication is 3 mg/kg on the first day, then 3 mg/kg (max 100 mg) daily for 7 days. However, if the child has renal impairment, the following advice needs to be heeded: usual initial dose, then halve subsequent doses if creatinine clearance < 50 mL/min per 1.73 m². How much fluconazole will a 4.5 kg (0.28 m²) baby have been administered after this course of therapy if the creatinine clearance is 5 mL/min?

A 48.75 mg
B 54 mg
C 60.75 mg
D 94.5 mg
E 108 mg

34 A syringe driver contains 15 mL diamorphine hydrochloride 4 mg/mL solution. The length of the syringe driver is 60 mm. What rate should the syringe driver be set at, so that the patient receives 5 mg/h of diamorphine hydrochloride?

A 3 mm/h
B 4 mm/h
C 5 mm/h
D 6 mm/h
E 7 mm/h

35 A 3-year-old girl has been prescribed ganciclovir (as the sodium salt) as maintenance therapy at a dose of 6 mg/kg daily on 5 days/week until she has adequate recovery of immunity after a transplantation. She weighs 12 kg and has normal renal function. For administration as an intravenous infusion the ganciclovir (as the sodium salt) powder is reconstituted with water for injections (500 mg/10 mL), then diluted to a concentration of 5 mg/mL with 0.9% sodium chloride, and the infusion then given over 1 hour. What flow rate is appropriate for this patient and how much ganciclovir (as the sodium salt) will she have been administered after 1 week?

A 0.24 mL/min and 360 mg
B 7.2 mL/min and 504 mg
C 18 mL/min and 360 mg
D 30 mL/min and 360 mg
E 30 mL/min and 504 mg

36 A patient is administered potassium chloride as a slow infusion over 150 min at a rate of 0.1 mmol potassium/kg per h. If 15 mmol potassium is delivered during the infusion what weight is the patient?

A 50 kg
B 55 kg
C 60 kg
D 65 kg
E 75 kg

37 The recommended oral dose for pericyazine for children aged between 1 and 12 years is initially 500 micrograms daily for 10-kg child, increased by 1 mg for each additional 5 kg to maximum total daily dose of 10 mg. Which of the following initial doses is within these guidelines?

A 0.25 mL pericyazine 10 mg/5 mL syrup daily for a 10 month old weighing 10 kg
B 0.5 mL pericyazine 10 mg/5 mL syrup daily for a 14 month old weighing 10 kg
C 1.75 mL pericyazine 10 mg/5 mL syrup daily for a 10 year old weighing 25 kg
D 2.5 mL pericyazine 10 mg/5 mL syrup daily for a 12 year old weighing 35 kg
E 7 mL pericyazine 10 mg/5 mL syrup daily for a 12 year old weighing 45 kg

38 A 9-year-old patient with asthma is being transferred from terbutaline sulphate 1.5 mg/5 mL syrup to terbutaline sulphate 5 mg tablets. The patient is currently taking 8 mL of the syrup three times a day. Which of the following is the most appropriate dosage as tablets for this patient? The tablets are scored and not coated.

A Half a tablet three times daily
B Half a tablet twice daily
C One tablet daily
D One tablet three times daily
E One tablet twice daily

39 A 6 year old is to be prescribed topiramate as monotherapy for partial seizures. This child weighs 20 kg and her consultant has decided to prescribe her drug according to a regimen of 0.5 mg/kg at night for 1 week, then increased in steps of 500 micrograms/kg at 1-week intervals, with the drug given twice daily. Her therapy is started on 1 August. Assuming that she tolerates her medication and the prescribed regimen is effective, what dose will she be receiving on 15 August?

    A   One 15 mg topiramate sprinkle capsule twice daily
    B   One 15 mg topiramate sprinkle capsule three times a day
    C   One 25 mg topiramate tablet daily
    D   One 25 mg topiramate sprinkle capsule twice daily
    E   One 50 mg topiramate tablet once daily

40 Following a medication review a patient currently being prescribed opioid analgesia is to have his analgesia changed. Previously the patient was taking 5.2 mg hydromorphone hydrochloride every 4 hours and now is to be prescribed oxycodone hydrochloride. Given that 1.3 mg hydromorphone hydrochloride is approximately equivalent to 5 mg oxycodone hydrochloride orally, and the patient takes the drug fully compliantly throughout the 24 hours of a day, which of the following dosage regimens is a suitable alternative for this patient?

    A   5 mg oxycodone hydrochloride capsules every 4 h
    B   20 mg oxycodone hydrochloride capsules every 6 h
    C   15 mL oxycodone hydrochloride 5 mg/5 mL liquid every 6 h
    D   3 mL oxycodone hydrochloride 10 mg/mL concentrate every 6 h
    E   20 mg oxycodone hydrochloride MR (modified-release) tablets every 12 h

41 A patient receiving palliative care has been recently changed from oral morphine sulphate solution to intramuscular 4-hourly injections of diamorphine hydrochloride. It has now been decided to change the analgesia to a 24-hourly subcutaneous infusion of diamorphine hydrochloride. The prescriber has authorised for any breakthrough pain to be managed by a subcutaneous injection of diamorphine hydrochloride, equivalent to one-sixth of the total 24-hour subcutaneous infusion dose. Given that the patient was receiving 20 mg diamorphine hydrochloride intramuscularly every 4 hours, which of the following is a suitable dose of diamorphine hydrochloride for any breakthrough pain?

A   3 mg
B   7 mg
C   13 mg
D   20 mg
E   30 mg

42 A 70-kg adult patient is being treated for iron poisoning. He is administered desferrioxamine mesilate initially at a dose of 12 mg/kg per h to be reduced by 25% after 6 h. How much desferrioxamine mesilate will this patient have received after 12 hours of therapy?

A   0.0882 g
B   0.882 g
C   63 g
D   6300 mg
E   8820 mg

Directions for Questions 43–54. For each numbered question select the one lettered option that is most closely related to it. Within the group of questions each lettered option may be used once, more than once, or not at all.

Questions 43–45 concern the following quantities:

A   0.75 g
B   0.787 g
C   0.882 g
D   7.55 g
E   7.875 g

Select, from A to E above, which is appropriate:

43 The amount of dimercaprol administered to a 75-kg patient for mercury poisoning when the following dosage regimen is prescribed: 3 mg/kg every 4 h over 2 days, three times a day on the third day, then twice daily for 10 days.

44 The amount of simeticone taken daily when 10 mL Altacite Plus suspension is taken twice daily and at bedtime. (Altacite Plus suspension: co-simalcite 125/500 [simeticone 125 mg, hydrotalcite 500 mg]/5 mL.)

45 The amount of simeticone administered to a baby when the maximum six doses of Dentinox colic drops is given to a baby for 7 consecutive days. Each dose contains 21 mg simeticone.

Questions 46–48 concern the following quantities:

    A   15
    B   60
    C   62.5
    D   115
    E   165

Select, from A to E above, which is appropriate:

---

46 The total number of millimoles of Na^+ contained within a 250 mL bottle of Gaviscon Advance suspension, given that there are 2.3 mmol Na^+ and 1 mmol K^+/5 mL.

47 The total number of millimoles K^+ consumed from 10 days' use of Fybogel Mebeverine granules at a dose of one sachet twice daily for 5 days and then an additional sachet taken daily on the remaining 5 days (contains 2.5 mmol K^+/sachet).

48 The total number of days therapy available within a 300 mL bottle of ranitidine (as hydrochloride) 75 mg/5 mL oral solution, when it is prescribed at a dose of 300 mg at night.

Questions 49–51 concern the following quantities:

    A   3.0 mL/min
    B   13.5 mL/h
    C   22.5 mL/min
    D   23.4 mL/min
    E   30 mL/h

Select, from A to E above, which is appropriate:

---

49 An appropriate initial intravenous infusion rate of enoximone when prescribed for an 83.5-kg patient at an initial dose of 90 micrograms/kg

per min. Enoximone is available as 5 mg/mL injections, which are diluted to a concentration of 2.5 mg/mL with 0.9% sodium chloride before administration.

50 An appropriate intravenous infusion rate of milrinone (as lactate) when prescribed for a 75-kg patient after surgery, at a dose of 600 ng/kg per min. Milrinone (as lactate) is available as 10 mL ampoules of concentration 1 mg/mL. These ampoules are diluted to a concentration of 200 micrograms/mL with 5% glucose before use.

51 An appropriate intravenous infusion rate of drug A when prescribed for a hospitalised 60-kg patient at a dose of 150 micrograms/kg over 20 min for an arrhythmia. In the hospital 10 mL ampoules of drug A 500 micrograms/mL are available. Before administration to this patient two of these ampoules are diluted in 500 mL 0.9% sodium chloride.

Questions 52–54 concern the following quantities:

    A   35
    B   48
    C   70
    D   140
    E   336

Select, from A to E above, which is appropriate:

52 The correct number of methotrexate 2.5 mg tablets to supply for a 9-year-old patient, weighing 28 kg and with a body surface area of 1.0 m², who is being maintained on an oral dose of methotrexate 15 mg/m² weekly to last her 8 weeks.

53 The number of 5 mg dexamfetamine sulphate tablets that a patient being treated for narcolepsy will use over the initial 4 weeks of therapy when prescribed as follows: 10 mg daily in two divided doses increased at weekly intervals by 10 mg daily to a maximum of 60 mg daily.

54 The correct number of etoposide 50 mg capsules to supply to a male patient, with a body surface area of 1.75 m², prescribed etoposide 200 mg/m² daily for 5 days.

Directions for Questions 55–60. The questions in this section are followed by three responses. **ONE** or **MORE** of the responses is (are) correct. Decide which of the responses is (are) correct. Then choose:

    A If 1, 2 and 3 are correct
    B If 1 and 2 only are correct
    C If 2 and 3 only are correct
    D If 1 only is correct
    E If 3 only is correct

Directions summarised:

A	B	C	D	E
1, 2, 3	1, 2 only	2, 3 only	1 only	3 only

55 A 65-kg patient is prescribed sodium nitroprusside for hypertensive crisis by intravenous infusion. The registrar has requested that the drug is prescribed initially as 1 microgram/kg per min, and then increased in steps of 500 ng/kg per min every 5 min up to a maximum of 8 micrograms/kg per min. If the infusion is commenced at 10.10am:

    1 At 10.13am 65 mg sodium nitroprusside will have been administered

    2 At 10.17am 0.52 mg sodium nitroprusside will have been administered

    3 At 10.21am the patient will be receiving the drug at a rate of 0.00013 g/min

56 Which of the following is (are) correct?

    1 A dose rate of 20 micrograms/min is equivalent to 1.2 mg/h

    2 A dose rate of 15 mg/h is equivalent to 0.000015 kg/h

    3 A dose rate of 10 drops/min is equivalent to 0.006 L/h given that 1 drop = 0.1 mL

57 Calcijex (calcitriol) injection is available as 1 mL ampoules available in two strengths: 1 microgram/mL and 2 micrograms/mL. The injection solution can be given orally.

    1 A 1-year-old girl, weighing 10 kg, is prescribed calcitriol orally at a dose of 20 ng/kg once daily for vitamin D-dependent

rickets. It is appropriate to give this girl 0.4 mL of the 1 microgram/mL injection solution daily

2   An 18-month-old girl, weighing 2 stone, is prescribed calcitriol orally at a dose of 15 ng/kg daily for hypophosphataemic rickets. It is appropriate to give this girl 0.25 mL of the 2 micrograms/mL injection solution daily. (1 stone ≈ 6.35 kg)

3   A 16-year-old boy, weighing 55 kg, is prescribed calcitriol orally at a dose of 0.001 mg daily for persistent hypocalcaemia. It is appropriate for this boy to take 0.5 mL of the 2 micrograms/mL injection solution daily

58 Epoetin beta has been prescribed for a range of indications for the following patients:

1   Mr B, weighing 75 kg, has been prescribed the drug at a dose of 20 units/kg three times weekly for 4 weeks. Over the 4 weeks Mr B will have taken 18 000 units epoetin beta

2   Catherine, weighing 60 kg, has recently had her dose increased to 80 units/kg three times weekly for 4 weeks. Each week Catherine will take 14 400 units epoetin beta

3   A 2-day-old neonate, weighing 1.25 kg, has been prescribed epoetin beta at a dose of 250 units/kg three times weekly. Each week this newborn will be given 937.5 units

59 Which of the following is (are) correct?

1   2 L of a solution is to be given to a patient over an 8-hour period. If 10 drops equal 0.5 mL the solution should be given at a rate of 100 drops/min

2   1 L of a solution is to be given to a patient over a 2-hour period. If one drop equals 0.1 mL the solution should be given at a rate of 25 drops/min

3   5 L of a solution is to be given to a patient over a 10-hour period. If one drop equals 0.2 mL the solution should be given at a rate of 2500 drops/h

60 Which of the following is (are) correct?

1   You receive a prescription for hydroxycarbamide 80 mg/kg every third day for the month of February, with the first dose to be taken on 3 February. The patient weighs 50 kg, so you should supply 72 hydroxycarbamide 500 mg capsules

2   At 9.45am a 1 L bag of 0.9% saline infusion is set up for a

patient at an administration rate of 1 mL/min. After $8\frac{1}{2}$ hours the doctor requests the flow rate to be increased to 90 mL/h. The bag will be due for replacement at 1am

3   An 11-year-old girl is prescribed Solvazinc effervescent tablets at a dose of one tablet three times a day. After the first week of compliant therapy she will have taken 9.45 g elemental zinc. Each Solvazinc effervescent tablet contains 125 mg zinc sulphate monohydrate (45 mg elemental zinc)

ANSWERS

1 E

Each dose of Mucogel suspension is 10 mL, so it contains 2 × 195 mg magnesium hydroxide

Each day Mrs A takes four doses, so she will have taken 20 doses in 5 days

Therefore she will have taken (20 × 2 × 195) mg = 7800 mg = 7.8 g.

So, the correct answer is E.

2 C

10 mg/kg twice daily for a 30-kg patient means that he will take (10 × 30 × 2) mg daily

After 4 weeks (28 days) the patient will have taken (10 × 30 × 2 × 28) mg = 16 800 mg

Each capsule contains 150 mg, so the patient will use (16 800/150) capsules in 4 weeks = 112.

Therefore, the correct answer is C.

3 A

Each day the patient will use 1.5 g twice daily = 3 g

Suspension strength is 1 g/5 mL, so the patient will use (3 × 5) mL daily

Each bottle contains (175/[3 × 5]) days = 11.66667, i.e. 11 complete days.

Therefore, the correct answer is A.

4 C

Adult dose: 1.5–3 mg two to three times daily

Elderly dose: 0.75–1.5 mg two to three times daily

A: (3 × 500) micrograms three times daily = 1.5 mg three times daily – appropriate

B: (2 × 500) micrograms three times daily = 1 mg three times daily – appropriate

C: (6 × 500) micrograms three times daily = 3 mg three times daily – not appropriate

D: (0.5 mL × 2 mg/mL) = 1 mg twice daily – appropriate

E: 1.5 mg three times daily – appropriate.

Therefore, the correct answer is C.

5 E
5 mg/kg twice daily for 18-kg child equates to $(5 \times 18 \times 2)$ mg daily = 180 mg daily
Epanutin suspension is 30 mg/5 mL, so patient needs $(180/30 \times 5)$ mL daily = 30 mL daily
October has 31 days, so in October the patient will use (31×30) mL = 930 mL.
Therefore, the correct answer is E.

6 E
Drug C dose: 4 mg/kg per h for 70 kg patient rate is 4×70 mg/h = 280 mg/h
Drug C available as 10 mg/2 mL solution, so rate is $(280/10) \times 2$ mL/h = 56 mL/h.
Therefore, the correct answer is E.

7 A
Fusidic acid dose: 500 mg three times daily $\times$ 10 days = 15 000 mg = 15 g = 0.015 kg.
Therefore, the correct answer is A.

8 A
Dose: 200 micrograms/m^2 daily in two doses, so single dose of 100 micrograms/m^2. For this patient this equates with 100×0.4 micrograms = 40 micrograms = 0.04 mg
Drug D liquid concentration is 0.1 mg/mL, so 0.04/0.1 mL = 0.4 mL.
Therefore, the correct answer is A.

9 B
Drug M dose is 7.5 mg/kg, so for a 10-kg patient dose this is 75 mg
Drug M available as 5 mg/mL, so 75/5 mL = 15 mL
Rate: 5 mL/min, so 15/5 min = 3 min.
Therefore, the correct answer is B.

10 D
Patient weight = 30 lb = 30×0.45 kg = 13.5 kg
Dose: 5 mg/kg four times daily for 7 days
Amount taken = $(5 \times 13.5 \times 4 \times 7)$ mg = 1890 mg = 1.89 g.
Therefore, the correct answer is D.

11 C
3 L = 3000 mL to be given over 2$^1/_2$-hour period, i.e. 150 min = 3000 mL/150 min
10 drops /1 mL therefore rate is ([3000 × 10] mL/150 min) = 200 drops/min.
Therefore, the correct answer is C.

12 A
Vial concentration is 75 mg/mL and 10 mL volume, so each vial contains 750 mg
750 mg/10 mL, so 75 mg in 1 mL, and 300 mg in 4 mL of 75 mg/mL
Needs to be diluted to 25 mg/mL before use, so a 1 in 3 dilution
1 in 3 dilution using 4 mL of original means total volume = 12 mL.
Therefore, the correct answer is A.

13 B
100 mg/mL, so 75 mg in 0.75 mL to be administered
U100 syringes, so 100 units/mL, so 0.75 mL delivered from (0.75 × 100) units = 75 units.
Therefore, the correct answer is B.

14 B
Dose: 4 mg/kg per day in three divided doses, so 4 × 75 mg daily in three divided doses = 300 mg daily in three divided doses
Each dose to be 100 mg = 5 × 20 mg capsules.
Therefore, the correct answer is B.

15 C
Has to be four times daily dosage interval, so B not suitable answer straight away
Baby weighs 18 kg, so recommended dosage is (3 × 18)–(5 × 18) daily in four divided doses = 54–90 mg daily in four divided doses = 13.5–22.5 mg four times daily, so 15 mg four times daily suitable.
Therefore, the correct answer is C.

16 A
5 mg/kg per day for a patient weighing 14 kg = 5 × 14 mg/day =70 mg daily = 70 000 micrograms.
Therefore, the correct answer is A.

17 B
Dose: 4 mg/kg daily in three divided doses. For this patient this means 4 ×
27 mg daily in three divided doses, so each individual dose is 36 mg
Suspension strength is 40 mg/5 mL; 1 mg in 5/40 mL; 36 mg in (5 × 36/40)
mL = 4.5 mL.
Therefore, the correct answer is B.

18 E
Oral daily dose: 12 mg/kg for 14 days for 80-kg patient; this is 12 × 80 mg
daily = 960 mg daily
Therefore over 14 days will use 960 × 14 mg = 13 440 mg
Drug D suspension is 30 mg/2 mL, so 1 mg in (2/30) mL and 13 440 mg in
(2 × 13 440/30) mL = 896 mL.
Therefore, the correct answer is E.

19 D
4 mg/mL suspension, so 12 mg in 3 mL
Therefore each dose is 3 mL four times daily
Daily going to need 3 × 4 mL = 12 mL
For 30 days going to need 12 × 30 mL = 360 mL.
Therefore, the correct answer is D.

20 A
Dose: 500 ng/kg per min for an 80-kg patient means 500 × 80 ng/min =
40 000 ng/min = 40 micrograms/min
Administered at concentration of 400 micrograms/mL, so 40 micrograms in
0.1 mL
Therefore, the IV rate should be 0.1 mL/min.
Therefore, the correct answer is A.

21 C
Dose: 6 mg/kg as Fiona weighs 6.25 kg will be given (6 × 6.25) mg for each
dose = 37.5 mg
Daily will receive 37.5 mg twice daily = 75 mg
Solution concentration: 5% w/v, so 5 g drug E in 100 mL solution
Therefore 1 g in 20 mL = 1000 mg in 20 mL = 1 mg in (20/1000) mL
75 mg required daily which is in (75 × 20/1000) mL = 1.5 mL.
Therefore, the correct answer is C.

22 E
Question states drug to be given three times daily, so answers C and D incorrect
Baby weighs 2.7 kg = 2700 g
Dose: 1 drop/450 g body weight three times daily
2700/450 = 6
Therefore dose is 6 drops three times daily.
Therefore, the correct answer is E.

23 A
Daily uses 8 g Solaraze gel, so over 60 days will use 480 g gel
Gel strength is 3%, so 3 g diclofenac sodium in 100 g gel and 3/100 g diclofenac sodium in 1 g gel. This means that 480 g contains (480 × 3/100) g diclofenac sodium = 14.4 g.
Therefore, the correct answer is A.

24 C
Patient weighs 70 kg, so standard dose to be used.
Treatment course:
2500 units
400 units/ h × 2 h = 800 units
300 units/h × 2 h = 600 units
200 units/h × 5 days = 200 × 24 × 5 units = 24 000 units
Total = 2500 +800 + 600 + 24 000 units = 27 900 units.
Formulated as 1250 units/mL, so will use (27 900/1250) mL = 22.32 mL.
Therefore, the correct answer is C.

25 C
Dose: 300 mg three times daily × 3 days = 2700 mg in total
Each sachet contains 600 mg, so over the 3 days will use 2700/600 sachets = 4.5 sachets
Each sachet contains 9 mmol sodium, so 4.5 sachets will contain 4.5 × 9 mmol = 40.5 mmol.
Therefore, the correct answer is C.

26 A
Ampoule strength is 50 mg/mL so each 2 mL dose contains 100 mg pethidine hydrochloride. Patient receives five doses, so will receive 100 × 5 mg pethidine hydrochloride.
Therefore, the correct answer is A.

27 D
Days 1–7: 5 mg morning
Days 8–14: 5 mg morning and night (doses over 5 mg given in two divided doses)
Days 15–21: 10 mg morning and 5 mg night – day 17 total daily dose is 15 mg
Days 22+: 10 mg twice daily – 5 mg = 10 drops – therefore 20 drops twice daily.
Therefore, the correct answer is D.

28 B
3 L over 4 h = 3000 mL over 4 × 60 min
Giving set delivers 2 drops/mL, so will deliver 2 × 3000 drops for 3000 mL = 6000 drops
Rate therefore: 6000 drops/240 min = (6000/240) drops/min = 25 drops/min.
Therefore, the correct answer is B.

29 E
4 mg/min × 30 min = 4 × 30 mg = 120 mg
2 mg/min × 2 h = 2 × 60 × 2 mg = 240 mg
1 mg/min × 10 h = 1 × 10 × 60 mg = 600 mg
Total drug given = 120 + 240 + 600 mg = 960 mg.
Therefore, the correct answer is E.

30 E
Drug dose: 5 micrograms/kg per min for 64 kg patient means (5 × 64) micrograms/min = 320 micrograms/min = 0.32 mg/min
Drug strength: 1.6 mg/mL = 1 mg in (1/1.6) mL, so 0.32 mg in (0.32/1.6) mL = 0.2 mL
Rate, therefore: 0.2 mL/min = (0.2 × 60) mL/h = 12 mL/h.
Therefore, the correct answer is E

31 C
1 in 10 000 means 1 g adrenaline (as acid tartrate) in 10 000 mL
Therefore 1 mL contains 1/10 000 g
Therefore 10 mL contains 10/10 000 g = 0.001 g = 1 mg.
The correct answer is, therefore, C.

32 C

1 mole NaCl = 23 + 35.5 g = 58.5 g

0.9% strength means 0.9 g NaCl in 100 mL solution = 9 g in 1 L

58.5 g = 1 mol

1 g = 1/58.5 mol

9 g = 9/58.5 mol ≈ 0.1538 mol ≈ 154 mmol.

Therefore, the correct answer is C.

33 C

First of all we need to compare the renal function for this child against the limit for changing the dose of the medication.

The limit is 50 mL/min per 1.73 m^2

For this child: he has a clearance of 5 mL/min, which is per 0.28 m^2 because we are told that this is the surface area for the child

Therefore, it is 5 mL/min per 0.28 m^2, which equates to (5/0.28) × 1.73 mL/min per m^2

= 30.89 mL/min per 1.73 m^2

This is below the limit of 50 mL/min per 1.73 m^2, so the child will receive the drug following the alternative dosing regimen

Dose received: initial dose of 3 mg/kg on day 1, then 1.5 mg/kg daily for 7 days

For 4.5-kg patient = (3 × 4.5) + (1.5 × 4.5 × 7) mg = 60.75 mg.

Therefore, the correct answer is C.

34 C

Solution concentration is 4 mg/mL; 15 mL of this solution contains 4 × 15 mg = 60 mg

Syringe driver length is 60 mm, so going to deliver 60 mg over length of 60 mm = 1 mg/mm

Rate required is 5 mg/h; this equates to 5 mm/h.

Therefore, the correct answer is C.

35 A

Dose of 6 mg/kg daily for a 12-kg patient – 72 mg daily

Rate of 72 mg/h = 72/60 mg/min = 1.2 mg/min

Strength of 5 mg/mL = 1 mg in 1/5 mL or 0.2 mL, so 1.2 mg is in 1.2 × 0.2 mL/min

= 0.24 mL/min

Total amount in 1 week = 72 × 5 mg; as only 5 days admin given = 360 mg.
Therefore, the correct answer is A.

36 C
0.1 mmol/kg per h is rate used.
150 min = 2.5 h
Making the patient weight = x kg
$0.1 \times x \times 2.5 = 15$
$0.25x = 15$
$x = 60$ kg.
Therefore, the correct answer is C.

37 C
Option A: child aged 10 months, so not within guidelines
Option B: weight 10 kg, so initial dose should be 500 micrograms; 0.5 mL
of 10 mg/5 mL = 1 mg
Option C: weight 25 kg, so initial dose should be 500 micrograms + ([25 –
10]/5) mg = 3.5 mg; 1.75 mL of 10 mg/5 mL = 3.5 mg
Option D: weight 35 kg, so initial dose should be 500 micrograms + ([35 –
10]/5) mg = 5.5 mg; 2.5 mL of 10 mg/5 mL = 5 mg
Option E: weight 45 kg, so initial dose should be 500 micrograms +
([45–10]/5) mg = 7.5 mg; 7 mL of 10 mg/5 mL = 14 mg.
Therefore, the correct answer is C.

38 A
8 mL of 1.5 mg/5 mL contains 8 × 1.5/5 mg = 2.4 mg
Daily dose is therefore 2.4 mg three times daily
2.5 mg ($^1/_2$ tablet) three times daily is the closest dose of those suggested.
Therefore, the correct answer is A.

39 A
1–7 August: 0.5 mg/kg at night
8–14 August: 0.5 mg/kg + 0.5 mg/kg (given twice daily)
15–21 August: 0.5 mg/kg + 1 mg/kg (given twice daily)
Therefore, on 15 August, girl taking 1.5 mg/kg in two divided doses. For a
20-kg patient this is (1.5 × 20)/2 mg twice daily = 15 mg twice daily.
Therefore, the correct answer is A.

40 D
5.2 mg hydromorphone hydrochloride every 4 hours = 5.2 × 6 doses in 24-h period = 31.2 mg
1.3 mg hydromorphone hydrochloride ≈ 5 mg oxycodone hydrochloride
31.2 mg hydromorphone hydrochloride ≈ 120 mg oxycodone hydrochloride
Option A: 5 mg × 6 doses = 30 mg
Option B: 20 mg × 4 doses = 80 mg
Option C: 15 mL × 5 mg/5 mL × 4 doses = 60 mg
Option D: 3 mL × 10 mg/mL × 4 doses = 120 mg
Option E: 20 mg × 2 doses = 40 mg.
Therefore, the correct answer is D.

41 D
20 mg every 4 h = 20 mg × 6 = 120 mg daily
Breakthrough dose = 1/6 of 120 mg = 20 mg.
Therefore, the correct answer is D.

42 E
0–6 hours 12 mg/kg per h → 12 × 6 × 70 mg = 5040 mg
6–12 hours 0.75 (12) mg/kg per h → 0.75 × 12 × 6 × 70 mg = 3780 mg
Total received after 12 h = 5040 mg + 3780 mg = 8820 mg.
Therefore, the correct answer is E.

43 E
2 days @ 3 mg/kg every 4 h = 3 × 75 × 6 × 2 mg = 2700 mg
1 day @ 3 mg/kg three times daily = 3 × 75 × 3 mg = 675 mg
10 days @ 3 mg/kg twice daily = 3 × 75 × 2 × 10 = 4500 mg
Total amount given = 2.7 g + 0.675 g + 4.5 g = 7.875 g.
Therefore, the correct answer is E.

44 A
125 mg simeticone per 5 mL
Daily takes 10 mL three times = 30 mL, so takes 30/5 × 125 mg = 750 mg = 0.75 g.
Therefore, the correct answer is A.

45 C
21 mg simeticone per dose

6 doses per day for 7 days = 42 doses
Therefore takes 882 mg simeticone = 0.882 g.
Therefore, the correct answer is C.

46 D
2.3 mmol Na$^+$/5 mL
Each 250 mL bottle contains 250/5 5 mL doses = 50 5 mL doses
Each bottle therefore contains 50 × 2.3 mmol Na$^+$ = 115 mmol Na$^+$
Therefore, the correct answer is D.

47 C
5 days: one sachet twice daily = 2.5 × 10 mmol K$^+$ = 25 mmol K$^+$
5 days: one sachet three times daily = 2.5 × 15 mmol K$^+$ = 37.5 mmol K$^+$
Over 10 days will take 25 + 37.5 mmol K$^+$ = 62.5 mmol.
Therefore, the correct answer is C.

48 A
Each dose is 300 mg at night
Strength is 75 mg/5 mL, so each dose is (300/75) × 5 mL = 20 mL
Each bottle contains 300 mL, which contains 300/20 mL = 15 doses = 15
days' therapy.
Therefore, the correct answer is A.

49 A
Dose: 90 micrograms/kg per min for this patient means 90 × 83.5
micrograms/min = 7515 micrograms/min = 7.515 mg/min
Given at strength of 2.5 mg/mL, so rate required is 7.515/2.5 mL/min ≈
3 mL/min.
Therefore, the correct answer is A.

50 B
Dose: 600 ng/kg per min for 75 kg = 600 × 75 ng/min = 45 000 ng/min =
45 micrograms/min
Given at strength of 200 micrograms/mL
Rate is therefore 45/200 mL/min = 0.225 mL/min = 13.5 mL/h.
Therefore, the correct answer is B.

51 D

Dose is 150 micrograms/kg over 20 min for 60-kg patient = 150 × 60 micrograms over 20 min = 9000 micrograms over 20 min = 9 mg over 20 min

Each ampoule is 500 micrograms/mL and 10 mL size, so contains 500 × 10 micrograms = 5000 micrograms = 5 mg

Two ampoules diluted in 500 mL, so 2 × 10 mL containing 10 mg diluted in 500 mL

The concentration being given is 10 mg in 520 mL = 10 mg/520 mL = 1 mg/52 mL

Rate is therefore 52 × 9 mL over 20 min = 468 mL/20 min = 23.4 mL/min.

Therefore, the correct answer is D.

52 B

Dose: 15 mg/m^2 for a patient with a body surface area (BSA) of 1 m^2 = 15 mg weekly × 8 weeks = 120 mg

Each tablet = 2.5 mg, so need 120/2.5 tablets = 48 tablets.

Therefore, the correct answer is B.

53 D

5 mg twice daily × 1 week = 14 tablets

10 mg twice daily × 1 week = 28 tablets

15 mg twice daily × 1 week = 42 tablets

20 mg twice daily × 1 week = 56 tablets

Total tablets used = 140 tablets.

Therefore, the correct answer is D.

54 A

Dose: 200 mg/m^2 for patient with BSA of 1.75 m^2 = 350 mg daily × 5 days = 1750 mg

Capsules each contain 50 mg, so need 1750/50 capsules = 35 capsules.

Therefore, the correct answer is A.

55 C

10.10–10.15am: 1 microgram/kg per min for 65 kg patient = 65 micrograms/min

10.15–10.20am: 1.5 micrograms/kg per min for 65 kg patient = 97.5 micrograms/min

10.20–10.25am: 2 micrograms/kg per min for 65 kg patient = 130 micrograms/min

1   At 10.13am will have 3 min of treatment given at 65 micrograms/min = 195 micrograms

       So 1 is false.

2   At 10.17am will have 5 min of treatment given at 65 micrograms/min and 2 min at 97.5 micrograms/min = 520 micrograms

       So 2 is true.

3   At 10.21am the rate is 130 micrograms/min = 0.13 mg/min = 0.00013 g/min

       So 3 is true.

Therefore, the correct answer is C.

56 B

1   20 micrograms/min = 20 × 60 micrograms/h = 1200 micrograms/h = 1.2 mg/h

       So 1 is true.

2   15 mg/h = 0.015 g/h = 0.000015 kg/h

       So 2 is true.

3   One drop = 0.1 mL, so 10 drops/min = 1 mL/min = 60 mL/h = 0.06 L/h

       So 3 is false.

Therefore, the correct answer is B.

57 E

1   Dose for 1-year-old girl is 20 ng/kg weighing 10 kg = 200 ng

       0.4 mL of 1 microgram/mL = 0.4 microgram

       So 1 is false.

2   1 stone = 6.35 kg, so 2 kg is 12.7 kg

       Dose for 18 month old is 15 × 12.7 ng = 190.5 ng

       0.25 mL × 2 micrograms/mL = 0.5 microgram

       So 2 is false.

3   Dose = 0.001 mg

       0.5 mL × 2 micrograms/mL = 1 microgram = 0.001 mg

       So 3 is true.

Therefore, the correct answer is E.

58 A

1   20 units/kg three times weekly × 4 weeks → 20 × 75 units × 3 × 4 = 18 000 units, so 1 is true.

2   80 units/kg three times weekly → 80 × 60 × 3 units = 14 400 units,
     so 2 is true.
3   250 units/kg three times weekly → 250 × 1.25 × 3 units = 937.5 units,
     so 3 is true.
Therefore, the correct answer is A.

59 E
1   2 L over 8 hours = 2000 mL/8 h = 250 mL/h
     10 drops = 0.5 mL, so 250 mL = 500 drops/h
     So 1 is false.
2   1 L over 2 h = 1000 mL/2 h = 500 mL/h
     25 drops/min = 2.5 mL/min = 1500 mL/h
     So 2 is false.
3   5 L over 10 h = 5000 mL/10 h = 500 mL/h
     2500 drops/h = 2500 × 0.2 mL/h = 500 drops/h,
     So 3 is true.
Therefore, the correct answer is E.

60 D
1   Doses on 3, 6, 9, 12, 15, 18, 21, 24 and 27 February, so nine doses
     to be given
     Dose: 80 mg/kg, so 80 × 50 mg = 4000 mg × 9 doses
     Need to supply (4000/500) × 9 capsules = 72 capsules
     So 1 is true.
2   9.45am infusion started at 1 mL/min, so 60 mL/h
     After $8^1/_2$ hours will have given 60 × $8^1/_2$ mL = 510 mL; this will be
     at 6.15pm
     Flow rate, now 90 mL/h, will give further 490 mL after 490/90 h =
     5.44 hours ≈ 5 h and 26 min; this will occur at about 11.41pm
     So 2 is false.
3   Each tablet contains 45 mg elemental Zn
     In 1 week will take 21 tablets, which contain 45 × 21 mg= 945 mg =
     0.945 g
     So 3 is false.
Therefore, the correct answer is D.

3 Pharmacokinetics

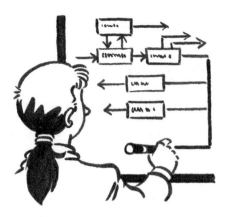

This chapter gives the reader an introduction to a wide range of applications of some pharmacokinetic principles. It does not, however, cover pharmacokinetics in depth and, if you believe that you need further 'in-depth' practice with pharmacokinetics, we suggest that you refer to some of the specialised texts that are on the market. Pharmacokinetics involves the use of many equations to which we introduce the reader in this chapter. It is important to understand how to manipulate formulae successfully before completing this chapter. The range of topics covered within our questions includes drug degradation, loading doses, renal clearance and serum concentrations. These questions can initially appear intimidating for a student; however, it is hoped that repeated practice will increase confidence and competence. In practice, drug doses often have to be adjusted according to altered renal clearance and reference may need to be made to specialised texts, e.g. Appendix 3 of the *British National Formulary* (BNF). We again suggest that you be completely familiar with the type of information included in your own recommended texts because this may be required in an open book calculation examination.

After completing the questions in this chapter you should be able to:

- understand the calculations that are required to identify the half-life of a drug
- calculate the creatinine clearance for individual patients
- use creatinine clearance to suggest the most appropriate dosage regimen of a drug
- estimate loading and maintenance doses.

QUESTIONS

Directions for Questions 1–42. Each of the questions or incomplete statements in this section is followed by five suggested answers. Select the best answer in each case.

1   Drug M with a half-life $(t_{1/2})$ of 45 min displays first-order kinetics, which means that the rate of change of drug concentration in the body by any process is directly proportional to the drug concentration remaining. Which of the following is the elimination rate constant (k_{el}) of drug M given that $k_{el} = 0.693/t_{1/2}$.

   A   1.54 min^{-1}
   B   0.0154 h^{-1}
   C   0.0154 min^{-1}
   D   0.0145 min^{-1}
   E   0.0145 h^{-1}

2   Miss A is given an intravenous dose of drug B and her peak serum level is found to be 20 mg/L. Given that 18 hours later her serum concentration is 2.5 mg/L, which of the following is the elimination half-life of drug B in this patient? (You may assume that the distribution is complete and that the elimination is described by a first-order process.)

   A   2 h
   B   4 h
   C   6 h
   D   8 h
   E   10 h

3   Brian, aged 76 and weighing 72 kg, requires a loading dose of drug C. Which of the following is the most suitable intravenous loading dose of drug C for Brian? (Volume of distribution $[V_D] = 4$ L/kg; therapeutic range 3–4 ng/mL.)

   A   500 micrograms
   B   750 micrograms
   C   1000 micrograms
   D   1250 micrograms
   E   1500 micrograms

4   A 54-year-old male patient with a body weight of 65 kg requires an oral loading dose of digoxin. You know that the volume of distribution (V_D) per kg body weight is 6 L, the salt factor (S) = 1 and the bioavailability (F) = 0.7. What dose should be used to achieve a target plasma concentration (C_p) of 1.25 micrograms/L?

$$\text{Loading dose} = \frac{(V_D \times C_p)}{(S \times F)}$$

  A   500 micrograms
  B   600 micrograms
  C   700 micrograms
  D   800 micrograms
  E   900 micrograms

5   Dan, who is 68 years old, has tonic–clonic seizures. As part of his clinical management plan it has been agreed between Dan, his consultant, and you, as his supplementary prescriber, to initiate him on levetiracetam. On checking Dan's case notes you see that his serum creatinine is 250 micromoles/L, and he weighs 65 kg.

$$\text{Creatinine clearance (mL/min)} = \frac{1.23 \times (140 - \text{age}) \times \text{weight (kg)}}{\text{serum creatinine (micromoles/L)}}$$

Guidance on prescribing of levetiracetam for tonic–clonic seizures with regard to renal function:

Creatinine clearance (mL/min)	Maximum daily dose (g)
> 80	3
50–80	2
30–50	1.5
< 30	1
< 10	Avoid use

Given Dan's renal function and using the provided prescribing guidance, which of the following is the maximum daily dose of levetiracetam that he should be prescribed?

  A   4 g
  B   3 g
  C   2 g
  D   1.5 g
  E   1 g

6   A woman is admitted to hospital after an accidental overdose of drug E. Upon hospital admission on 1 September at 1.00am her plasma concentration of drug E is 240 micrograms/mL. Given that the half-life $(t_{1/2})$ of drug E is 16 h, what will be her plasma concentration of drug E at 3.00am on 3 September? (You may assume that the distribution is complete and the elimination is described by first-order process.)

    A   150 micrograms/mL
    B   120 micrograms/mL
    C   90 micrograms/mL
    D   60 micrograms/mL
    E   30 micrograms/mL

7   A patient is taken to the accident and emergency department (A&E) of his local hospital by his brother after an overdose of an antibiotic. The drug's half-life $(t_{1/2})$ is 6.5 h. The tests carried out upon admission show a toxic plasma concentration of 88 micrograms/mL. How long will it take for the plasma concentration to reach a non-toxic concentration of 5.5 micrograms/mL? (You may assume that the distribution is complete and that the elimination is described by a first-order process.)

    A   13 h
    B   19.5 h
    C   22.75 h
    D   26 h
    E   32.5 h

8   A 55-year-old man is admitted to hospital after a drug overdose. The drug's half-life $(t_{1/2})$ is 10 h. A toxic plasma concentration of 108 micrograms/mL is recorded. After 60 h, what would you expect the plasma concentration of the drug to be? (You may assume that the distribution is complete and that the elimination is described by a first-order process.)

    A   6750 ng
    B   3375 ng
    C   1687.500 ng
    D   843.750 ng
    E   421.875 ng

9   You are the renal pharmacist in your hospital and the junior house officer (JHO) consults you about prescribing valaciclovir for herpes zoster to a patient, Mr Foster, under his care. Mr Foster is 82 years of

age and weighs 62 kg, has a body surface area of 1.67 m² and a serum creatinine concentration of 0.3 micromoles/mL. Taking into account his renal function and the guidance that you have on valaciclovir prescribing, which dose is appropriate for you to advise the JHO to prescribe?

$$\text{Creatinine clearance (mL/min)} = \frac{1.23 \times (140 - \text{age}) \times \text{weight (kg)}}{\text{serum creatinine (micromoles/L)}}$$

Local prescribing on valaciclovir for herpes zoster:

Creatinine clearance (mL/min)	Daily dose
> 30	1 g three times daily
15–30	1 g every 12 h
< 15	1 g every 24 h

    A   1 g four times daily
    B   1 g three times daily
    C   1 g every 12 h
    D   1 g every 24 h
    E   0.5 g every 24 h

10 Gregory, who is 44 years old, has partial seizures. His doctor has decided to prescribe levetiracetam (Keppra) for him and asks you to advise on a suitable dose. On checking Gregory's case notes you see that his serum creatinine is 450 micromoles/L and his weight 62 kg. Given the information below, which is a suitable dosage of Keppra for Gregory?

$$\text{Creatinine clearance (mL/min)} = \frac{1.23 \times (140 - \text{age}) \times \text{weight (kg)}}{\text{serum creatinine (micromoles/L)}}$$

Guidance on prescribing of levetiracetam for partial seizures with regard to renal function:

Creatinine clearance (mL/min)	Maximum daily dose (MDD) (g)
> 80	3
50–80	2
30–50	1.5
< 30	1
< 10	Avoid use

Levetiracetam should be prescribed at a dosage interval of twice daily.

A   500 mg Keppra tablet morning and night
B   500 mg Keppra tablet in the morning and 750 mg Keppra tablet at night
C   750 mg Keppra tablet morning and night
D   1 g Keppra tablet morning and night
E   10 mL of Keppra oral solution (100 mg/mL) morning and night

11 A patient is given an intravenous dose of drug H and her peak serum level is found to be 12 micrograms/mL; 12 hours later her serum concentration is 0.75 mg/L. What is the elimination half-life ($t_{1/2}$) of drug H in this patient? (You may assume that the distribution is complete and that the elimination is described by a first-order process.)

A   2 h
B   3 h
C   4 h
D   5 h
E   6 h

12 A 54-year-old male patient weighing 65 kg requires a loading dose of drug K to treat an infection. Which is a suitable intravenous loading dose of drug K for this patient to achieve a concentration between 7 and 9 mg/L? (Drug K volume of distribution $[V_D] = 0.25$ L/kg.)

A   75 mg
B   100 mg
C   125 mg
D   150 mg
E   175 mg

13 Drug N with an elimination rate constant (k_{el}) of 0.21 h^{-1} displays first-order kinetics. Given that $k_{el} = 0.693/t_{1/2}$, which of the following is the half-life ($t_{1/2}$) of drug N?

A   3.3 min
B   198 s
C   198 h
D   33 min
E   198 min

14 Using the following equation for females, decide which of the suggestions is the most appropriate estimate of creatinine clearance (Cl_{Cr}) for Linda, who is aged 60, weighs 70 kg and has a serum creatinine of 175 micromoles/L:

$$Cl_{Cr} \text{ (mL/min)} = \frac{1.04 \times (140 - \text{age}) \times \text{weight (kg)}}{\text{serum creatinine (micromoles/L)}}$$

- **A** 39.36 mL/min
- **B** 36.17 mL/min
- **C** 33.28 mL/min
- **D** 32 mL/min
- **E** 30.11 mL/min

15 The Jelliffe equation can be used to estimate creatinine clearance (Cl_{Cr}) in units of mL/min per 1.73 m². For males:

$$Cl_{Cr} = \frac{98 - 0.8 \times (\text{patient's age in years} - 20)}{\text{serum creatinine (mg/dL)}}$$

Using the Jelliffe equation, what is the estimated creatinine clearance for Arthur, aged 88 years, who has a serum creatinine of 2 mg/dL, weighs 70 kg and has a body surface area of 1.85 m²?

- **A** Approximately 12.60 mL/min
- **B** Approximately 21.80 mL/min
- **C** Approximately 22.72 mL/min
- **D** Approximately 23.31 mL/min
- **E** Approximately 25.20 mL/min

16 A 30-year-old woman weighing 11 stone has received a single intravenous 10 mg dose of a benzodiazepine. A blood sample taken after this administration shows a plasma concentration of 40 micrograms/100 mL of the drug. What is the volume of distribution (V_D) of this drug, given that 1 stone ≈ 6.35 kg and $V_D = \text{dose}/C_p^{0}$.

- **A** 0.25 L
- **B** 1.75 L
- **C** 2.5 L
- **D** 17.5 L
- **E** 25 L

17 What is the elimination rate constant (k_{el}) for drug B, which has an elimination half-life ($t_{1/2}$) of 7 h, given that $k_{el} = 0.693/t_{1/2}$? (You may assume that the elimination is described by a first-order process.)

- **A** 0.099 h^{-1}
- **B** 0.99 h^{-1}
- **C** 1.98 h^{-1}

    D   2.97 h^{-1}
    E   5.94 h^{-1}

18 The volume of distribution (V_D) of drug C was determined to be 20 L. What would be the expected drug plasma concentration immediately after an intravenous dose of 2 mg is given to a 70-kg male patient? V_D = dose/C_p^0.

    A   0.01 microgram/dL
    B   0.1 microgram/dL
    C   1 microgram/dL
    D   10 micrograms/dL
    E   100 micrograms/dL

19 Doreen has been given a 600 mg dose of drug E while in hospital. The elimination half-life of drug E is 8 h and it follows first-order kinetics. How much of this drug will remain in her system 48 h after administration, assuming that complete absorption and distribution have occurred?

    A 937.5×10^{-10} kg
    B 937.5×10^{-9} kg
    C 937.5×10^{-8} kg
    D 937.5×10^{-7} kg
    E 937.5×10^{-6} kg

20 Which is the best estimate of the plasma concentration of drug F when 2 g is given by intravenous bolus to a 31-year-old patient weighing 10 stone, 12 lb. The volume of distribution of drug F for this patient is 0.9 L/kg? (1 stone ≈ 6.35 kg; 1 lb ≈ 0.45 kg; V_D = dose/C_p^0.)

    A   2.22 mg/L
    B   32.25 mg/L
    C   35.00 mg/L
    D   42.34 mg/L
    E   46.67 mg/L

21 Which of the following is the best estimate of the creatinine clearance (Cl_{Cr}) for Grace, a 74-year-old renal patient, who weighs 66 kg and has a serum creatinine of 125 micromoles/L? For females:

$$Cl_{Cr} \text{ (mL/min)} = \frac{1.04\ (140 - \text{age}) \times \text{weight (kg)}}{\text{serum creatinine (micromoles/L)}}$$

A 0.362 L/h
B 2.091 L/h
C 2.175 L/h
D 34.848 L/h
E 36.242 L/h

22 The clearance of phenytoin from the body is calculated using the Michaelis–Menten model. Clearance of phenytoin:

$$Cl_{phenytoin} = \frac{V_{max}\ (mg/day)}{K_m\ (mg/L) + serum\ concentration\ (mg/L)}$$

where V_{max} is the maximum metabolic capacity (mg/day) and K_m is the plasma concentration at which the rate of metabolism is half the maximum (mg/L).

Assuming that V_{max} is 7 mg/kg per day and K_m is 4 mg/L, which of the following is the best estimate of phenytoin clearance in Mr H who is 71 years old, weighs 72 kg and has a serum concentration of 20 mg/L?

A 20 L/day
B 21 L/day
C 22 L/day
D 23 L/day
E 24 L/day

23 Phenytoin has a narrow therapeutic index and hence small changes in drug absorption may result in a marked change in plasma concentration. Individual maintenance doses should be calculated for patients to maintain patient safety. The following equation can be used for this purpose:

Maintenance dose (mg) =

$$\frac{(V_{max} \times serum\ concentration)}{S \times F \times (K_m\ [mg/L] + serum\ concentration\ [mg/L])}$$

Isobel, a 63 kg woman newly diagnosed with epilepsy, requires a serum concentration of 18 mg/L for optimum response. Isobel is to be prescribed phenytoin as capsules; the maximum metabolic capacity (V_{max}) is 7 mg/kg per day and the plasma concentration at which the rate of metabolism is half the maximum (K_m) is 4 mg/L. Which dose is a suitable maintenance dose for Isobel, given that the bioavailability (F) of phenytoin capsules is 1 and the salt factor (S) is 0.92?

 A 300 mg
 B 350 mg
 C 400 mg
 D 450 mg
 E 500 mg

24 Jim, a 54-year-old inpatient on the coronary care ward, is to be prescribed digoxin elixir. The JHO on the ward asks for your advice about a suitable loading dose for Jim, who weighs 75 kg. What is a suitable loading dose for you to recommend for prescribing to Jim? You have access to the following information:
Loading dose = $(V_D \times C_p)/(S \times F)$
Volume of distribution (V_D) = 7 L/kg
Target concentration (C_p) = 1.2 ng/mL
Bioavailability (F) = 0.77
Salt factor (S) = 1

 A 10.5 mL digoxin, 50 micrograms/mL elixir
 B 12 mL digoxin, 50 micrograms/mL elixir
 C 16.5 mL digoxin, 50 micrograms/mL elixir
 D 20 mL digoxin, 50 micrograms/mL elixir
 E 25 mL digoxin, 50 micrograms/mL elixir

25 Mrs K is to be given gentamicin for an infection and the target concentration that you, as the independent prescriber, want to achieve is 8 mg/L. Mrs K weighs 65 kg. Given the information below, what is a suitable loading dose for you to prescribe?
Loading dose = $(V_D \times C_p)/(S \times F)$
Volume of distribution (V_D) = 0.25 L/kg
Bioavailability (F) = 1
Salt factor (S) = 1

 A 120 mg
 B 130 mg
 C 140 mg
 D 150 mg
 E 160 mg

26 The amount of drug required to keep a steady serum concentration of the drug is the maintenance dose. The maintenance dose can be defined as:
Maintenance dose (mg/h) = amount of drug removed/$(S \times F)$
Liam is to be given drug M every 8 h, which has a clearance rate of 6

L/h and a serum concentration of 27 mg/L. What is a suitable maintenance dose for you, as the ward clinical pharmacist, to recommend to the medical team involved in the care of Liam, assuming that the bioavailability and salt factor are both 1?

    A   162 mg
    B   216 mg
    C   612 mg
    D   962 mg
    E   1296 mg

27 A patient has been given a 200 mg dose of carbamazepine tablets. A peak serum concentration of 4 mg/L is recorded after the administration. Given the following equation and that the bioavailability (F) and salt factor (S) are both equal to 1, which is the best estimate of the patient's volume of distribution?

Dose $= (V_D \times C_p)/(S \times F)$

    A   50 L
    B   100 L
    C   200L
    D   400 L
    E   800 L

28 Arnold has been started on a new drug to control his recent respiratory symptoms. This drug is completely renally excreted from the body. He is given a dose of 250 mg and, when his urine is analysed, it is found that 220 mg of the drug is present in the urine. What is the best estimate of the bioavailability (F) of this drug given the information below?

Amount of drug reaching systemic circulation $= F \times S \times$ dose

    A   0.79
    B   0.88
    C   0.97
    D   1.06
    E   1.14

29 Beth has a theophylline serum concentration of 96 mg/L following a period of taking her theophylline tablets four times a day instead of twice daily. Given that the half-life of theophylline is 8 h, how long will it take for her serum concentration to reach a target concentration of 12 mg/L? (You may assume that the distribution is complete and that the elimination is described by a first-order process.)

A 4 h
B 8 h
C 16 h
D 24 h
E 32 h

30 Cathal, who is 54 years old, has mild renal impairment and weighs 63 kg. Before his doctor is willing to recommend a dose of venlafaxine for his depression, he wants to calculate his creatinine clearance. What is the best estimate of Cathal's creatinine clearance given the equation below and that his serum creatinine is 175 micromoles/L?

$$\text{Creatinine clearance (mL/min)} = \frac{1.23 \times (140 - \text{age}) \times \text{weight (kg)}}{\text{serum creatinine (micromoles/L)}}$$

A 29.22 mL/min
B 30.96 mL/min
C 32.64 mL/min
D 34.10 mL/min
E 38.08 mL/min

31 Diane, aged 84 years, is to be given an intravenous loading dose of digoxin. Upon admission to hospital Diane's weight was recorded in her notes as 59 kg. The JHO on the ward asks for your advice about a suitable loading dose for Diane, to achieve a serum concentration of 0.002 mg/L. Which of the following is a suitable loading dose for you to recommend to the JHO?
You have access to the following information:
Loading dose = $(V_D \text{ [L]} \times C_p)/(S \times F)$
Volume of distribution (V_D) = 7.3 L/kg
Target concentration (C_p) = 0.002 mg/L
Bioavailability (F) = 1
Salt factor (S) = 1

A 0.08614 microgram
B 0.8614 microgram
C 8.614 micrograms
D 86.14 micrograms
E 861.4 micrograms

32 What loading dose of intravenous aminophylline would be suitable for a 60-kg male patient requiring a serum concentration of 15 mg/L?
You have access to the following information:

Loading dose = $(V_D \text{ [L]} \times C_p)/(S \times F)$
Volume of distribution (V_D) = 0.5 L/kg
Target concentration (C_p) = 0.002 mg/L
Bioavailability (F) = 1
Salt factor (S) = 0.8

A   0.0075 microgram
B   0.075 microgram
C   0.75 microgram
D   7.5 micrograms
E   75 micrograms

33 Edward is a 61-year-old male patient, weighing 62 kg, who has been
given a 300 mg intravenous dose of gentamicin for an infection 1 hour
previously. The volume of distribution of gentamicin in this patient is
0.25 L/kg and the bioavailability (F) and salt factor (S) are both 1. (You
may assume that there is negligible elimination during this 1-hour
period.) Which of the following is the best estimate of the gentamicin
peak serum concentration in Edward?
Dose = $(V_D \text{ [L]} \times C)/(S \times F)$

A   1.20 mg/mL
B   4.84 mg/L
C   19.35 micrograms/mL
D   20.67 micrograms/mL
E   21.19 mg/L

34 What is the creatinine clearance of a 72-year-old male patient who
weighs 61 kg and has a measured serum creatinine of 160 micro-
moles/L?

$$\text{Creatinine clearance (mL/min)} = \frac{1.23 \times (140 - \text{age}) \times \text{weight (kg)}}{\text{serum creatinine (micromoles/L)}}$$

A   1.91 L/h
B   2.62 L/h
C   3.94 L/h
D   25.93 L/h
E   31.89 L/h

35 Which loading dose of digoxin tablets would you recommend for a 72
kg male patient requiring a serum concentration of 1 microgram/L?
Loading dose = $(V_D \text{ [L]} \times C_p)/(S \times F)$
V_D = volume of distribution = 7.3 L/kg

C_p = serum concentration
S = salt factor = 1
F = bioavailability = 0.7

    A   62.5 micrograms
    B   125 micrograms
    C   250 micrograms
    D   500 micrograms
    E   750 micrograms

36 Mrs Fletcher is admitted to accident and emergency with fast atrial fibrillation and requires digoxin therapy. She is 75 kg in weight. What oral loading dose would you recommend to the prescribing doctor who contacts you about this patient explaining he is aiming to achieve a serum concentration of 1.5 micrograms/L? Your hospital policy on the prescribing of digoxin recommends that you assume the volume of distribution to be 7 L/kg, the salt factor to be 1 and the bioavailability of digoxin tablets to be 0.7 and of digoxin elixir to be 0.77. The loading dose can be given in divided doses over 24 hours or as a single dose.
Loading dose = $(V_D \text{ [L]} \times C_p)/(S \times F)$

    A 3×250 microgram digoxin tablets over 24 h in divided doses
    B 2×250 microgram digoxin tablet and 1×125 microgram tablet over 24 h in divided doses
    C 4×250 microgram digoxin tablet and 1×125 microgram tablet over 24 h in divided doses
    D   15 mL digoxin elixir 50 micrograms/L as a single dose
    E   35 mL digoxin elixir 50 micrograms/L over 24 h as divided doses 6 h apart

37 The dosage schedule for Timentin depends on the patient's creatinine clearance (Cl_{Cr}) as follows:
Cl_{Cr} > 60 mL/min: 3.2 g every 6 h
Cl_{Cr} 30–60 mL/min: 3.2 g every 8 h
Cl_{Cr} 10–30 mL/min: 1.6 g every 8 h
Cl_{Cr} < 10 mL/min: 1.6 g every 12 h
Miss H is 34 years old, weighs 51 kg, and has a serum creatinine concentration (S_{cr}) of 250 micromoles/L. The formula for Cl_{Cr} in females is:

$$Cl_{Cr} \text{ (mL/min)} = \frac{1.04 \times (140 - \text{age}) \times \text{weight (kg)}}{\text{serum creatinine (micromoles/L)}}$$

Which of the following dosage regimens would be suitable for Miss H?

    A   3.2 g every 4 h
    B   3.2 g every 6 h
    C   3.2 g every 8 h
    D   1.6 g every 8 h
    E   1.6 g every 12 h

38 An 81-kg patient requires oral theophylline for his chronic asthma. Which of the following dosage regimens of a 12-hourly modified-release theophylline preparation would provide a steady-state plasma concentration (C_{ss}) between 10 and 20 mg/L, assuming that oral bioavailability (F) is 1, the salt factor (S) is 1, his clearance (Cl) is 36.67 mL/min and the volume of distribution (V_D) is 0.5 L/kg?
Maintenance dose = $(C_{ss} \times Cl \times$ dosage interval$)/(F \times S)$

    A   60 mg every 12 h
    B   125 mg every 12 h
    C   175 mg every 12 h
    D   250 mg every 12 h
    E   350 mg every 12 h

39 The dosage schedule for drug K depends on the patient's creatinine clearance (Cl_{Cr}) as follows:
Cl_{Cr} > 50 mL/min: 6 mg/kg every 6 h
Cl_{Cr} 30–50 mL/min: 4 mg/kg every 6 h
Cl_{Cr} 15–30 mL/min: 4 mg/kg every 8 h
Cl_{Cr} 10–15 mL/min: 2 mg/kg every 12 h
Cl_{Cr} < 10 mL/min: 1 mg/kg every 12 h
Mr L is 35 years old, weighs 75 kg and has a serum creatinine concentration of 80 micromoles/L. The formula for creatinine clearance (Cl_{Cr}) is:

$$Cl_{Cr} \text{ (mL/min)} = \frac{1.23 \times (140 - \text{age}) \times \text{weight (kg)}}{\text{serum creatinine (micromoles/L)}}$$

Which of the following is a suitable dosage regimen for Mr L?

    A   450 mg every 6 h
    B   300 mg every 6 h
    C   300 mg every 8 h
    D   150 mg every 12 h
    E   75 mg every 12 h

40 Which of the following is the amount of drug M available for absorption after a night-time dose of one 250 mg tablet, given that the bioavailability of drug M tablets is 0.8?

    A   50 mg
    B   75 mg
    C   100 mg
    D   200 mg
    E   250 mg

41 An 8-year-old child is having his Lanoxin formulation changed from
    elixir to tablets due to a manufacturing problem with the elixir. The
    child is currently taking a dose of 1.3 mL of 50 micrograms/mL elixir
    twice daily. Given that the bioavailability of the tablets is 63% and the
    elixir is 75%, which of the following is a suitable alternative dosage
    regimen? (Digoxin can be given as a once or twice daily dose for
    children between the ages of 5 and 10 years.)

    A   125 microgram Lanoxin tablet twice daily
    B   62.5 microgram Lanoxin-PG tablet twice daily
    C   1 × 125 microgram Lanoxin and $^1/_2$ × 62.5 microgram
        Lanoxin-PG tablet daily
    D   250 microgram Lanoxin tablet daily
    E $1^1/_2$ 125 microgram Lanoxin tablets daily

42 While in hospital a patient has been receiving ranitidine as an
    intravenous injection of 50 mg every 6 h. This patient is being
    discharged from hospital and the doctor has contacted you in the
    pharmacy to recommend a bioequivalent dose of ranitidine 100 mg/5 mL
    oral solution. Knowing that the bioavailability of ranitidine oral
    solution is 50%, which of the following is a suitable dose for you to
    recommend?

    A   2 mL twice daily
    B   5 mL twice daily
    C   10 mL twice daily
    D   15 mL twice daily
    E   20 mL twice daily

Directions for Questions 43–54. For each numbered question select the
one lettered option that is most closely related to it. Within the group of
questions each lettered option may be used once, more than once, or not
at all.

Questions 43–45 concern the following quantities:

    A 5 L
    B 12 L
    C 37.5 L
    D 54 L
    E 60 L

Select, from A to E above, which is appropriate:

43 The apparent volume of distribution (V_D) when a 450 mg intravenous dose of drug N produces an immediate blood concentration of 7.5 micrograms/mL.
V_D can be defined as: $V_D = D/C_p$, in which D = total amount of drug in the body and C_p = plasma concentration of drug.

44 The apparent volume of distribution (V_D) when a 0.75 kg intravenous dose of drug P produces an immediate blood concentration of 20 g/L.

45 The apparent volume of distribution (V_D) when a 900 microgram intravenous dose of drug Q produces an immediate blood concentration of 1.8×10^{-7} g/mL.

Questions 46–48 concern the following quantities:

    A 3.338 mg
    B 5.000 mg
    C 8.924 mg
    D 11.679 mg
    E 13.125 mg

Select, from A to E above, which is appropriate:

46 The total amount of drug R present in the body 2 h after an intravenous injection, assuming that the apparent volume of distribution is 211 mL/kg. Drug R has been given to this patient, who weighs 71 kg, 2 h ago, and now has a drug R blood concentration of 50 micrograms/mL.
V_D can be defined as: $V_D = D/C_p$ in which D = total amount of drug in the body and C_p = plasma concentration of drug.

47 The amount of drug S that will be left in the body after 15 h, given that the half-life of drug S is 3 h and the initial dose given is 420 mg. (You may assume that the elimination process follows first-order kinetics.)

48 An appropriate intravenous loading dose of drug T for Victor. Victor is aged 77 and weighs 73 kg. The volume of distribution is 6 L/kg and the acceptable therapeutic concentration range is 10–20 micrograms/L.

Questions 49–51 concern the following quantities:

    A   1 h
    B   3 h
    C   6 h
    D   9 h
    E   12 h

Select, from A to E above, which is appropriate:

---

49 The half-life $(t_{1/2})$ of drug W, knowing that the plasma concentration of the drug is 300 mg/L at 5am and 37.5 mg/L at 11pm on the same day. (You may assume that the drug displays first-order kinetics.)

50 The half-life of drug X, which displays first-order kinetics and has an elimination rate constant (k_{el}) of 0.01155 min^{-1}, given that $k_{el} = 0.693/t_{1/2}$.

51 The length of time that it will take for the plasma concentration to decrease from 800 micrograms/mL per kg to 0.625 g/L in a 50 kg patient, given that the half-life of the drug is 30 min and the drug displays first-order elimination kinetics.

Questions 52–54 concern the following quantities:

    A   0.75 mg/mL
    B   15.38 mg/L
    C   17 micrograms/mL
    D   54 mg/L
    E   75 mg/mL

Select, from A to E above, which is appropriate:

52 The plasma concentration of drug Z in Mr A at 5.00pm on 15 March. Following an accidental overdose Mr A was admitted to hospital at 9.00pm on 14 March when his plasma concentration of drug Z was found to be 2400 mg/mL. The half-life of drug Z is 4 h. (You may assume that the distribution is complete and that the elimination is described by a first-order process).

53 The expected drug plasma concentration of drug B immediately after an intravenous dose of 200 mg is given to a 65-kg female patient. You know that the volume of distribution (V_D) of drug B is 0.2 L/kg and that $V_D = \text{dose}/C_p^0$.

54 The best estimate of the plasma concentration of drug C, when 0.004 kg is given by intravenous bolus to a 20-year-old patient weighing 9 stone, 2 lb. The volume of distribution of drug C for this patient is 4 L/kg? (1 stone $\approx$ 6.35 kg; 1 lb $\approx$ 0.45 kg; $V_D = \text{dose}/C_p^0$.)

Directions for Questions 55–60. The questions in this section are followed by three responses. **ONE** or **MORE** of the responses is (are) correct. Decide which of the responses is (are) correct. Then choose:

A   If 1, 2 and 3 are correct
B   If 1 and 2 only are correct
C   If 2 and 3 only are correct
D   If 1 only is correct
E   If 3 only is correct

Directions summarised:

A	B	C	D	E
1, 2, 3	1, 2 only	2, 3 only	1 only	3 only

55 C_p^0 is the initial plasma concentration of a drug following an initial dose. C_p^0 is dependent upon the dose and the apparent volume of distribution (V_D) of the drug such that:
$$V_D = \text{dose}/C_p^0$$

   1   A patient received a single intravenous dose of 200 mg drug A that produced an immediate blood concentration of 5 micrograms/mL. The V_D is therefore 40 L

2   Bob is given 0.15 g drug C, which has a V_D of 30 L. The immediate blood concentration would be 5 g/L

3   If C_p^0 after a dose of a drug is 4 mg/L and V_D is 32 L, the dose given is 8 mg

56 Following drug administration the amount of the dose that reaches the systemic circulation depends on the dose given, the bioavailability (*F*) of the drug and the salt factor (*S*). This relationship can be demonstrated by this equation:

Amount of drug reaching systemic circulation = $F \times S \times$ dose

Tegretol tablets (carbamazepine) have a bioavailability of 1 (available as 100 mg, 200 mg and 400 mg tablets).

Tegretol Retard tablets (carbamazepine) have a bioavailability of 0.85 (available as 200 mg and 400 mg modified-release tablets).

1   1200 mg carbamazepine is systemically absorbed in a day when a dose of 1 × 400 mg Tegretol tablet is taken three times a day

2   1020 mg carbamazepine is systemically absorbed in a day when a dose of 600 mg Tegretol Retard is taken twice daily

3   A patient being transferred from Tegretol tablets at a dose of 700 mg daily (400 mg in morning, 200 mg at lunchtime and 100 mg at teatime) to Tegretol Retard would be appropriately changed to 400 mg Tegretol Retard morning and night to maintain approximately constant levels of the drug in the systemic circulation

57 Drug D has a clearance rate of 0.02 L/min.

1   If initially the serum concentration of drug D is 6 mg/L after 12 h the concentration will be decreased by 86.4 mg

2   If initially the serum concentration of drug D is 0.8 g/L after 3 h the concentration will be decreased by 0.00288 kg

3   If the serum concentration of drug D has decreased by 10 mg after 6 h the initial concentration was 3 mg/L

58 A 53-year-old woman with epilepsy, weighing 56 kg, has been taking 150 mg phenytoin capsules daily to control her condition. Plasma concentration of phenytoin should be in the range 10–20 mg/L for optimum response from the drug. However, during a recent outpatient review, it was discovered that her plasma concentration was only 6 mg/L.

1 Given that the bioavailability (*F*) of phenytoin capsules is 1, the salt factor (*S*) is 0.92 and the plasma concentration at which the rate of metabolism is half the maximum (K_m) is 4 mg/L, the maximum metabolic capacity (V_{max}) in this patient would be 7 mg/kg per day

Maintenance dose (mg/day) = V_{max} × serum concentration/{S × F × (K_m [mg/L] + serum concn [mg/L])}

2 To achieve a serum concentration of 12 mg/L for this patient, her daily dose should be adjusted to 250 mg/day

3 To achieve a serum concentration of 15 mg/L for this patient, it would be appropriate to adjust her phenytoin daily dose to 200 mg

59 Gerald is admitted onto the coronary care ward where you are the clinical ward-based pharmacist. Gerald has fast atrial fibrillation and requires digoxin therapy. The ward policy for the prescribing of digoxin, which you co-authored with the ward consultant, includes the following information on the prescribing of digoxin:

Serum concentration aim for 1–2 micrograms/L

Salt factor = 1

Bioavailability = 0.7

Creatinine clearance (Cl_{Cr}) (mL/min) =

$$\frac{1.23 \times (140 - \text{age}) \times \text{weight (kg)}}{\text{serum creatinine (micromoles/L)}}$$

In a patient without heart failure:

Digoxin clearance (mL/min) = (0.8 × weight [kg]) + Cl_{Cr}

In a patient with congestive heart failure:

Digoxin clearance (mL/min) = (0.33 × weight [kg]) + (0.9 × Cl_{Cr})

Maintenance dose (micrograms) = (clearance rate × concentration × dosage interval)/(S × F)

The case notes of Gerald record the following information:

Sex: male

Age: 60

Weight: 80 kg

History of heart failure: none

Serum creatinine: 175 micromoles/L

Using the information above, apply the following to Gerald:

1 His creatinine clearance is 35 mL/min

2 His digoxin clearance is 45 mL/min

3 250 micrograms is a suitable maintenance dose

60 A patient is currently receiving drug A by intravenous injection while in hospital. Before discharge of this patient from hospital you discuss with the senior house officer (SHO) alternative routes of administration and the doses that would be appropriate for these different formulations.

Currently the patient is receiving drug A as an injection of 200 mg daily. Drug A is also available as 25 mg tablets, which have a bioavailability (*F*) of 0.65, and 25 mg/5 mL syrup, with a bioavailability of 0.8. The salt factor (*S*) for all these formulations is 1.

Amount of drug reaching systemic circulation = $F \times S \times$ dose

1 Following a dose of one 25 mg tablet of drug A, 16.25 mg drug A reaches the systemic circulation

2 Following a 50 mL daily dose of drug A syrup, 200 mg drug A is available for absorption

3 It would be appropriate to prescribe this patient drug A at a daily dose of 60 mL drug A syrup to implement a 20% increase in the current intravenous dose that he is receiving

ANSWERS

1 C
k_{el} = 0.693/45 min = 0.0154 min^{-1}
Therefore, the correct answer is C.

2 C
Peak is 20 mg/L, so after one half-life $(t_{1/2})$ concentration will be 10 mg/L, after another reduces to 5 mg/L, and then after a third $t_{1/2}$ reduces to a serum concentration of 2.5 mg/L
Therefore, $3 \times t^{1/2} = 18$ h
And each $t_{1/2} = 6$ h.
Therefore, the correct answer is C.

3 C
Volume of distribution (V_D) = 4 L/kg, so for a 72-kg patient = 4×72 L = 288 L
Therapeutic range = 3–4 ng/mL, so for a patient with a V_D of 288 L want to have a dose of $(3 \times 288 \times 1000)$–$(4 \times 288 \times 1000)$ ng
= 864 000–1152 000 ng
= 864–1152 micrograms.
Therefore the correct answer is C.

4 C
Loading dose (micrograms) = $(6 \text{ L} \times 65 \times 1.25 \text{ micrograms/L})/(1 \times 0.7)$
≈ 696.43 micrograms
≈ 700 micrograms.
Therefore, the correct answer is C.

5 E
Creatinine clearance (mL/min) = $(1.23 \times [140 - 68] \times 65)/250$
≈ 23.021 mL/min
The maximum daily dose is therefore 1 g because creatinine clearance < 30 mL/min but > 10 mL/min.
Therefore, the correct answer is E.

6 E
Plasma concentration decreases by half within each half-life of 16 h:
1.00am 1 September 240 micrograms/mL

5.00pm 1 September 120 micrograms/mL
9.00am 2 September 60 micrograms/mL
1.00am 3 September 30 micrograms/mL
Therefore, the correct answer is E.

7 D
Each $t_{1/2}$ = 6.5 h, over which time the plasma concentration will reduce by a half:
$88 \rightarrow 44 \rightarrow 22 \rightarrow 11 \rightarrow 5.5$
Therefore will take four half-lives to reduce from 88 micrograms/mL to 5.5 micrograms/mL
$t_{1/2}$ = 6.5 h, so will take 4×6.5 h = 26 h.
Therefore, the correct answer is D.

8 C
Each $t_{1/2}$ = 10 h, so after 60 h six half-lives will have passed, and the plasma concentration of the drug will have halved six times:
$108 \rightarrow 54 \rightarrow 27 \rightarrow 13.5 \rightarrow 6.75 \rightarrow 3.375 \rightarrow 1.6875$
Therefore, after 60 h the plasma concentration = 1.6875 micrograms/mL = 1687.5 ng.
Therefore, the correct answer is C.

9 D
Creatinine clearance (mL/min) = (1.23 × [140 – 82] × 62 [kg])/(0.3 × 1000 [micromoles/L])
≈ 14.74 mL/min
< 15 mL/min
Therefore, dose should be 1.5 g every 24 h.
So, the correct answer is D.

10 A
Creatinine clearance (mL/min) = (1.23 × [140 – 44] × 62 [kg])/450 micromoles/L ≈ 16.269 mL/min
= < 30 mL/min but > 10 mL/min, so MDD = 1 g
A–E all show drug frequency of twice daily, so no answer can be ruled out at this stage:
Option A: MDD = 1 g
Option B: MDD = 1250 mg
Option C: MDD = 1500 mg

Option D: MDD = 2 g
Option E: MDD = 10 × 100 mg × 2 = 2000 mg.
Therefore, the correct answer is A.

11 B
Peak serum level = 12 micrograms/mL
After 12 h, serum level = 0.75 mg/L
First of all need to have both concentrations in the same units
Peak serum level = 12 micrograms/mL
After 12 h, serum level = 0.75/1000 mg/mL = 0.00075 mg/mL = 0.75 micrograms/mL
12 → 6 → 3 → 1.5 → 0.75
Therefore, four half-lives have passed for serum concentration to reduce from 12 to 0.75 micrograms/mL
These four half-lives have taken 12 h, so each $t_{1/2}$ lasts 3 h.
Therefore, the correct answer is B.

12 C
Drug K is being administered intravenously, so the bioavailability and salt factor of the drug do not have to be considered.
Volume of distribution = 0.25 L/kg; for this patient weighing 65 kg this equates to 0.25 × 65 L = 16.25 L
Target concentration = 7–9 mg/L
As V_D = 16.25 L, the target concentration range is (7 × 16.25)–(9 × 16.25) mg = 113.75–146.25 mg
125 mg is the only suggested answer within this range.
Therefore, the correct answer is C.

13 E
$k_{el} = 0.693/t_{1/2}$, so $k_{el} \times t_{1/2} = 0.693$ and $0.21 \ h^{-1} \times t_{1/2} = 0.693$
$t_{1/2}$ (h) = 0.693/0.21 = 3.3 h
= 3.3 × 60 min = 198 min.
Therefore, the correct answer is E.

14 C
Cl_{Cr} (mL/min) = (1.04 × [140 – 60] × 70 [kg])/175 (micromoles/L)
= 33.28 mL/min.
Therefore, the correct answer is C.

15 D

$$Cl_{Cr} = \frac{98 - 0.8 \times (\text{patient's age in years} - 20)}{\text{serum creatinine (mg/dL)}}$$

$Cl_{Cr} = (98 - 0.8 \times [88 - 20])/2$
$Cl_{Cr} = 21.8$ mL/min per 1.73 m²
$Cl_{Cr} = (21.8/1.73)$ mL/min per m²
$Cl_{Cr} = (21.8 \times 1.85/1.73)$ mL/min for Arthur
$Cl_{Cr} \approx 23.31$ mL/min.
Therefore, the correct answer is D.

16 E

$V_D = \text{dose}/C_p^0$
Dose = 10 mg
Dose in milligrams, so need to convert C_p^0 to milligrams
Answers for V_D given in litres, so best to convert C_p^0 to litres now before doing the calculation
$C_p^0 = 40$ micrograms/100 mL = 0.04 mg/100 mL = 0.4 mg/L
$V_D = 10$ mg/0.4 mg/L = 25 L.
Therefore, the correct answer is E.

17 A

$k_{el} = 0.693/7$ h = 0.099 h⁻¹
Therefore, the correct answer is A.

18 D

$V_D = \text{dose}/C_p^0$
20 L = 2 mg/C_p^0
$C_p^0 = 2/20$ mg/L = 0.1 mg/L
Answers given as micrograms/dL so need to convert 0.1 mg/L into these units
0.1 mg/L = 100 micrograms/L = 10 micrograms/dL.
Therefore, the correct answer is D.

19 C

48 h/8 h = 6, so six half-lives have occurred during 48 h:
600 mg → 300 mg → 150 mg → 75 mg → 37.5 mg → 18.75 mg → 9.375 mg
After 48 h the amount of drug E left is 9.375 mg
9.375 mg = 0.009375 g = 0.000009375 kg = 937.5 × 10⁻⁸ kg.
Therefore, the correct answer is C.

20 B

First of all need to convert patient weight from imperial to metric:

Weight = 10 stone, 12 lb

1 stone = 6.35 kg, 1 lb = 0.45 kg, so this patient weights ([10 × 6.35] + [12 × 0.45]) kg = 68.9 kg

Volume of distribution = 0.9 L/kg, so 0.9 L/kg × 68.9 kg = 62.01 L

$V_D = \text{dose}/C_p^0$

$V_D/\text{dose} = 1/C_p^0$

$V_D \times C_p^0 = \text{dose}$

$C_p^0 = \text{dose}/V_D$

$C_p^0 = 2/62.01$ g/L

= 0.03225 g/L

= 32.25 mg/L.

Therefore, the correct answer is B.

21 C

$$Cl_{Cr} \text{ (mL/min)} = \frac{1.04 \, (140 - 74) \times 66 \text{ (kg)}}{125 \text{ (micromoles/L)}}$$

= 36.242 mL/min

Answers given in litres per hour so need to convert to these units

Cl_{Cr} (L/h) = 36.242 × 60 mL/h = 2.175 L/h.

Therefore, the correct answer is C.

22 B

Clearance of phenytoin $(Cl_{phenytoin})$ =

$$\frac{V_{max} \text{ (mg/day)}}{K_m \text{ (mg/L)} + \text{serum concentration (mg/L)}}$$

$Cl_{phenytoin}$ = 7 × 72 (mg/day)/4 (mg/L) + 20 (mg/L)

= 504/24 L/day = 21 L/day.

Therefore, the correct answer is B.

23 C

Maintenance dose (mg) = (7 × 63 × 18)/(0.92 × 1 × [4 + 18])

= 392.19 mg

In practice this dose would be given as 400 mg.

Therefore, the correct answer is C.

24 C

Loading dose = $(V_D \times C_p)/(S \times F)$

$$\text{Loading dose (micrograms)} = \frac{V_D \text{ (L)} \times C_p \text{ (microgram/L)}}{S \times F}$$

C_p = 1.2 ng/mL = 1.2 micrograms/L
V_D = 7 L/kg for 75-kg patient = (7 × 75) L = 525 L
Loading dose (micrograms) = (525 × 1.2)/(0.77 × 1)
= 818.18 micrograms
Elixir strength is 50 micrograms/mL, so 818.18 micrograms in 818.18/50
mL = 16.36 mL
In practice, the closest dose that could be given is 16.5 mL.
Therefore, the correct answer is C.

25 B
Loading dose (mg) = (0.25 × 65 × 8)/(1 × 1)
= 130 mg gentamicin.
Therefore, the correct answer is B.

26 E
Maintenance dose (mg/h) = amount of drug removed/$(S \times F)$

$$\text{Maintenance dose (mg)} = \frac{\text{clearance rate} \times \text{concentration} \times \text{dosage interval}}{S \times F}$$

= (6 L/h × 27 mg/L × 8 h)/(1 × 1)
= 1296 mg every 8 h.
Therefore, the correct answer is E.

27 A
Dose = $(V_D \times C_p)/(S \times F)$
200 mg = $(V_D \times 4 \text{ mg/L})/(1 \times 1)$
200 mg = $V_D \times 4$ mg/L
V_D = 200 mg/4 mg/L
= 50 L.
Therefore, the correct answer is A.

28 B
If drug completely eliminated by the kidneys will assume that 220 mg is the
amount of the 250 mg dose that reaches the systemic circulation
Amount of drug reaching systemic circulation = $F \times S \times$ dose
220 mg = $F \times 1 \times 250$ mg
F = 220/250
= 0.88.
Therefore, the correct answer is B.

29 D

$t_{1/2}$ = 8 h, so the serum concentration will reduce by 50% every 8 h
96 mg/L → 48 mg/L → 24 mg/L → 12 mg/L
Serum concentration will have decreased to 12 mg/L after three half-lives,
so over a period of 3 × 8 h = 24 h.
Therefore, the correct answer is D.

30 E

$$\text{Creatinine clearance (mL/min)} = \frac{1.23 \times (140 - \text{age}) \times \text{weight (kg)}}{\text{serum creatinine (micromoles/L)}}$$

= (1.23 × [140 − 54] × 63)/175
= 38.0808 mL/min ≈ 38.08 mL/min.
Therefore, the correct answer is E.

31 E

Loading dose = $(V_D \times C_p)/(S \times F)$
Loading dose (mg) = (7.3 L/kg × 59 kg × 0.002 mg/L)/(1 × 1)
= 0.8614 mg
= 861.4 micrograms.
Therefore, the correct answer is E.

32 E

Loading dose = ([0.5 × 60] L × 0.002 mg/L)/(0.8 × 1)
= 0.075 mg = 75 micrograms.
Therefore, the correct answer is E.

33 C

Dose = $(V_D \, [L] \times C)/(S \times F)$
300 mg = (0.25 L/kg × 62 kg × C)/(1 × 1)
C (mg/L) = 300/(0.25 × 62)
19.35 mg/L = 19.35 micrograms/mL.
Therefore, the correct answer is C.

34 A

Creatinine clearance (mL/min) = (1.23 × [140 − age] × weight [kg])/serum
creatinine (micromoles/L)
= (1.23 × [140 − 72] × 61 [kg])/160 (micromoles/L)
= 31.89 mL/min
= 31.89 × 60 mL/h = 1913.27 mL/h
= 1.91 L/h.
Therefore, the correct answer is A.

35 E
Loading dose = $(V_D \times C_p)/(S \times F)$
Loading dose (micrograms) = $([7.3 \times 72]$ L $\times$ 1 microgram/L)/1 $\times$ 0.7
= 750.86 micrograms
In practice the most suitable dose is 750 micrograms.
Therefore, the correct answer is E.

36 C
Loading dose = $(V_D \times C_p)/(S \times F)$
Loading dose for tablets = $(7 \times 75 \times 1.5)/0.7$ = 1125 micrograms
Loading dose for elixir = $7 \times 75 \times 1.5/0.77$ = 1022.73 micrograms
A: 3×250 micrograms = 750 micrograms over 24 h (tablet)
B: 2×250 micrograms + 125 micrograms = 625 micrograms over 24 h (tablet)
C: 4×250 micrograms + 125 micrograms = 1125 micrograms over 24 h (tablet)
D: 15 mL of digoxin 50 micrograms/mL elixir = 750 micrograms (elixir)
E: 35 mL of digoxin 50 micrograms/mL elixir = 1750 micrograms (elixir).
Therefore, the correct answer is C.

37 D

$$\text{Creatinine clearance (mL/min)} = \frac{1.04 \times (140 - \text{age}) \times \text{weight (kg)}}{\text{serum creatinine (micromoles/L)}}$$

= $(1.04 \times [140 - 34] \times 51)/250$
= 22.49 mL/min
Cl_{Cr} is between 10 and 30 mL/min, so the suitable dosage regimen is 1.6 g every 8 h.
Therefore, the correct answer is D.

38 E

$$\text{Maintenance dose} = \frac{C_{ss} \times Cl \times \text{dosage interval}}{F \times S}$$

Cl = 36.67 mL/min = 2200 mL/h = 2.2 L/h
Maintenance dose for concn of 10 mg/L = (10 mg/L $\times$ 2.2 L/h $\times$ 12 h)/ (1×1)
Maintenance dose (mg) = $10 \times 2.2 \times 12$
= 264 mg every 12 h
Maintenance dose for concn of 20 mg/L = 20 mg/L $\times$ 2.2 L/h $\times$ 12 h
Maintenance dose (mg) = 528 mg every 12 h

Therefore the maintenance for this patient needs to be within range 264–528 mg every 12 h.
Therefore, the correct answer is E.

39 A

$$\text{Creatinine clearance (mL/min)} = \frac{1.23 \times (140 - 35) \times 75}{80}$$

= (1.23 × 105 × 75)/80 mL/min
= 121.08 mL/min
Creatinine clearance is normal (> 50 mL/min), so the dosage regimen that should be followed is 6 mg/kg every 6 h
For a 75-kg patient this equates to (6 × 75) mg every 6 h
= 450 mg every 6 h.
Therefore, the correct answer is A.

40 D

A bioavailability of 0.8 indicates that 80% of the dose of drug M will be available for absorption
Amount available for absorption = 80% × 250 mg = 200 mg.
Therefore, the correct answer is D.

41 C

First, calculate the amount of bioavailable digoxin that the child is receiving from the Lanoxin elixir:
1.3 mL twice daily × 50 micrograms/mL = 50 × 1.3 × 2 micrograms daily
= 130 micrograms daily
75% of this dose is bioavailable = 0.75 × 130 micrograms = 97.5 micrograms.
Second, need to calculate the dose of Lanoxin tablets that will make 97.5 micrograms of digoxin bioavailable:
The bioavailability of Lanoxin tablets = 63% of dose
x micrograms Lanoxin tablets release 0.63x micrograms digoxin
x micrograms Lanoxin tablets release 97.5 micrograms digoxin
so 0.63x = 97.5
and x = 154.76 micrograms.
Therefore, the aim is to have 154.76 micrograms daily of Lanoxin tablets, but only available as 62.5, 125 and 250 microgram tablets; it is not going to be possible in practice to give this exact dose.

A: 250 micrograms daily
B: 125 micrograms daily
C: 156.25 micrograms daily
D: 250 micrograms daily
E: 187.5 micrograms daily.
Therefore, the correct answer is C.

42 C
When ranitidine given as an intravenous injection it is 100% bioavailable:
Intravenous dose: 50 mg every 6 h
So 200 mg bioavailable within 24 h
Therefore want 200 mg to be bioavailable from the oral dose
Bioavailability of oral solution is 50%, so need to take (200/50%) mg = 400 mg
Oral solution concentration is 100 mg/5 mL, so 400 mg available in 20 mL
Therefore the correct answer is C.

43 E
D = 450 mg = 450 000 micrograms
C_p = 7.5 micrograms/mL = 7500 micrograms/L
$V_D = D/C_p$
V_D (L) = 450 000 micrograms/7500 micrograms/L
V_D = 60 L.
Therefore, the correct answer is E.

44 C
D = 0.75 kg = 750 g
C_p = 20 g/L
$V_D = D/Cp$
V_D (L) = 750/20 = 37.5 L.
Therefore, the correct answer is C.

45 A
D = 900 micrograms
C_p = 1.8×10^{-7} g/mL = 0.18 micrograms/mL = 180 micrograms/L
$V_D = D/C_p$
V_D = 900/180 L = 5 L.
Therefore, the correct answer is A.

46 A

V_D= 211 mL/kg = 0.211 L/kg

For a 71-kg patient = 0.211 × 71 L = 14.981 L

C_p = 50 micrograms/mL = 50 000 micrograms/L = 50 mg/L

$V_D = D/C_p$

14.981 = 50/C_p

C_p = 50/14.981 = 3.338 mg.

Therefore, the correct answer is A.

47 E

The half-life is 3 h, so every 3 h the amount of drug present will decrease by 50%

During a period of 15 h five half-life periods each of 3 h will have passed

420 mg → 210 mg → 105 mg → 52.5 mg → 26.25 mg → 13.125 mg

Therefore, the correct answer is E.

48 B

Drug given intravenously, so the bioavailability of the drug does not have to be taken into account.

Loading dose = V_D × C_p

= 6 L/kg × 10 micrograms/L

= 6 L/kg × 73 kg × 10 micrograms/L

= 4380 micrograms = 4.38 mg

Loading dose = V_D × C_p

= 6 L/kg × 20 micrograms/L

= 6 L/kg × 73 kg × 20 micrograms/L

= 8760 micrograms = 8.76 mg

Therefore the loading dose should be in the range 4.38–8.76 mg.

Therefore, the correct answer is B.

49 C

$t_{1/2}$ = the length of time it takes for drug concentration to halve

300 mg/L → 150 mg/L → 75 mg/L → 37.5 mg/L

Therefore three half-lives have occurred during the time interval from 5am to 11pm

There is a time period of 18 hours

$t_{1/2}$ = 18/3 h = 6 h.

Therefore, the correct answer is C.

50 A
$k_{el} = 0.01155$ min$^{-1} = 0.693/t_{1/2}$
0.01155 min$^{-1} \times t_{1/2} = 0.693$
$t_{1/2} = 0.693/0.01155$ min $= 60$ min $= 1$ h.
Therefore, the correct answer is A.

51 B
Need to have both concentrations in the same units, so first will convert the initial concentration of 800 micrograms/mL per kg to a concentration of g/L:
800 micrograms/mL per kg for a 50-kg patient $= 800 \times 50$ micrograms/mL
$= 40\ 000$ micrograms/mL $= 40$ mg/mL $= 40\ 000$ mg/L $= 40$ g/L
Over each 30 min the drug concentration will reduce by 50%:
40 g/L $\rightarrow$ 20 g/L $\rightarrow$ 10 g/L $\rightarrow$ 5 g/L $\rightarrow$ 2.5 g/L $\rightarrow$ 1.25 g/L $\rightarrow$ 0.625 g/L
Therefore six half-lives will have passed for this concentration change to have occurred, and so the total time is 6×30 min $= 3$ h.
Therefore, the correct answer is B.

52 E
Plasma concentration decreases by half within each half-life of 4 h
21:00 on 14 March to 17:00 on 15 March is a 20-hour time period
Each half-life lasts 4 hours, so this time interval includes five half-lives
The concentration will decrease as follows:
9.00pm 14 March: 2400 mg/mL
1.00am 15 March: 1200 mg/mL
5.00am 15 March: 600 mg/mL
9.00am 15 March: 300 mg/mL
1.00pm 15 March: 150 mg/mL
5.00pm 15 March: 75 mg/mL.
Therefore, the correct answer is E.

53 B
$V_D = \text{dose}/C_p^{\ 0}$
$(0.2 \text{ L/kg} \times 65 \text{ kg}) = 200 \text{ mg}/C_p^{\ 0}$
$13 \text{ L} = 200 \text{ mg}/C_p^{\ 0}$
$200/13 \text{ mg/L} = C_p^{\ 0}$
$C_p^{\ 0} = 15.38 \text{ mg/L}$.
Therefore, the correct answer is B.

54 C
Patient's weight $= 9$ stone, 2 lb $= (9 \times 6.35) + (2 \times 0.45) = 58.05$ kg
$V_D = \text{dose}/C_p^{\ 0}$

$4 \text{ L/kg} \times 58.05 \text{ kg} = 0.004 \text{ kg}/C_p^0$

$232.2 \text{ L} = 4 \text{ g}/C_p^0$

$C_p^0 = 4/232.2 \text{ g/L}$

$= 0.017 \text{ g/L}$

$= 0.017 \text{ g/1000 mL}$

$= 17 \text{ mg/1000 mL}$

$= 17\,000 \text{ micrograms/1000 mL}$

$C_p^0 = 17 \text{ micrograms/mL.}$

Therefore, the correct answer is C.

55 D

1   $V_D = \text{dose}/C_p^0$
    $V_D = 200 \text{ mg/5 micrograms/mL}$
    $= 200 \text{ mg/5 mg/L}$
    $= 40 \text{ L}$

2   $V_D = \text{dose}/C_p^0$
    $30 \text{ L} = 0.15 \text{ g}/C_p^0$
    $C_p^0 = 0.15 \text{ g/30 L}$
    $= 0.005 \text{ g/L}$

3   $V_D = \text{dose}/C_p^0$
    $32 \text{ L} = \text{dose}/4 \text{ mg/L}$
    $\text{Dose} = 32 \text{ L} \times 4 \text{ mg/L}$
    $= 128 \text{ mg.}$

Therefore, 1 is true and 2 and 3 are false, so the correct answer is D.

56 A

1   Carbamazepine is not formulated as a salt within Tegretol, so the salt factor does not have to be considered
    Amount of drug reaching systemic circulation = $F \times S \times \text{dose}$
    $= 1 \times (400 \times 3) \text{ mg}$
    $= 1200 \text{ mg.}$

2   Amount of drug reaching systemic circulation = $F \times S \times \text{dose}$
    $= 0.85 \times (600 \times 2) \text{ mg}$
    $= 1020 \text{ mg.}$

3   When taking Tegretol at dose of 700 mg daily:
    Amount of drug reaching systemic circulation = $F \times S \times \text{dose}$
    $= 1 \times 700 \text{ mg} = 700 \text{ mg}$
    Therefore when transferred, want to maintain 700 mg as the amount of carbamazepine absorbed
    Amount of drug reaching systemic circulation = $F \times S \times \text{dose}$

700 mg = 0.85 × dose
Dose = 823.53 mg
Tegretol Retard at dose of 400 mg twice daily is the closest dose that can be given.
1, 2 and 3 all true, so the correct answer is A.

57 B

1   Clearance rate = 0.02 L/min = 0.02 × 60 L/h = 1.2 L/h
       After 12 h, therefore, 12 × 1.2 L will be cleared = 14.4 L
       Each litre contains 6 mg/L, so will clear 14.4 × 6 mg = 86.4 mg.

2   Clearance rate = 1.2 L/h
       After 3 h will have cleared 3 × 1.2 L = 3.6 L
       Concn = 0.8 g/L, so will clear 0.8 × 3.6 g over 3 h = 2.88 g = 0.00288 kg.

3   Clearance rate = 1.2 L/h
       After 6 h will have cleared 6 × 1.2 L = 7.2 L
       If lost 10 mg within 7.2 L, the initial concentration would be 10/7.2 mg/L = 1.39 mg/L.

Overall 1 and 2 correct but 3 false, so the correct answer is B.

58 E

1   Maintenance dose (mg/day) =

$$\frac{V_{max} \times \text{serum concentration}}{S \times F \times (K_m \,[\text{mg/L}] + \text{serum concentration [mg/L]})}$$

       150 (mg/day) = $(V_{max} \times 6 \text{ mg/L})/\{0.92 \times 1 \times (4 \,[\text{mg/L}] + 6 \,[\text{mg/L}])\}$
       150 (0.92 × [4 + 6])/6 = V_{max} mg/day
       V_{max} (mg/day) = 230 mg/day
       Patient weighs 56 kg, so this is 230/56 mg/kg per day = 4.107 mg/kg per day.

2   Maintenance dose (mg/day) =

$$\frac{V_{max} \times \text{serum concentration}}{S \times F \times (K_m \,[\text{mg/L}] + \text{serum concentration [mg/L]})}$$

       = 230 mg/day × 12 mg/L/{0.92 × 1 × (4 [mg/L] + 12 [mg/L])}
       = 2760/14.72 = 187.5 mg.

3   Maintenance dose (mg/day) =

$$\frac{V_{max} \times \text{serum concentration}}{S \times F \times (K_m \,[\text{mg/L}] + \text{serum concentration [mg/L]})}$$

       = 230 mg/day × 15 mg/L/{0.92 × 1 × (4 [mg/L] + 15 [mg/L])}
       = 3450/17.48 mg = 197.37 mg

In practice this would be given as 200 mg daily.
Overall 1 and 2 are false and 3 is true, so the overall answer is E.

59 E

1   Creatinine clearance (Cl_{cr}) (mL/min) $= \dfrac{1.23 \times (140 - 60) \times 80}{175}$

    Cl_{cr} (mL/min) = 44.98 mL/min.

2   Patient has no history of heart failure, so:
    Digoxin clearance (mL/min) = $(0.8 \times$ weight [kg]$) + Cl_{cr}$
    $= (0.8 \times 80) + 44.98$
    $= 108.98$ mL/min.

3   Digoxin clearance = 108.98 mL/min = 6538.8 mL/h = 6.54 L/h
    Maintenance dose (micrograms) = (clearance rate × concn × dosage interval)/$(S \times F)$
    = (6.54 L/h × 1 microgram/L × 24 h)/(0.7 × 1)
    = 224.23 micrograms for concn of 1 microgram/L
    Maintenance dose (micrograms) = (clearance rate × concn × dosage interval)/$(S \times F)$
    = (6.54 × 2 × 24)/(0.7 × 1)
    = 448.46 micrograms for concn of 1 microgram/L
Maintenance dose must then be within range 224.23–448.46 micrograms.
Overall, 1 and 2 are false and 3 is true, so the correct answer is E.

60 A

1   Amount of drug reaching systemic circulation = $F \times S \times$ dose
    $= 0.65 \times 1 \times 25$ mg
    $= 16.25$ mg.

2   Amount of drug reaching systemic circulation = $F \times S \times$ dose
    $= 0.8 \times 1 \times 50/5 \times 25$ mg
    $= 200$ mg.

3   Amount of drug reaching systemic circulation = $F \times S \times$ dose
    As an injection currently receiving 200 mg daily, so 200 mg reach systemic circulation. A 20% increase on dose would increase daily dose to 240 mg
    Amount of drug reaching systemic circulation = $F \times S \times$ dose
    Need to calculate the amount of drug reaching systemic circulation from 60 mL syrup and compare this with 240 mg calculated above
    Amount of drug reaching systemic circulation = $0.8 \times 1 \times 60/5 \times 25$
    $= 240$ mg.
Overall, answers 1, 2 and 3 are all true, so the correct answer is A.

4 Formulation and dispensing

This chapter introduces the user to calculations that are involved in the extemporaneous formulation and dispensing of a wide range of products. There are important concepts within these questions that are valuable and must be understood to gain a level of competence within this area of pharmaceutical practice. One of these is the different strengths of medicinal waters, e.g. chloroform water double-strength, single-strength and concentrate, in particular how the strength of each relates to the others, which links to the concept of dilutions in formulation. The pharmacist must always be aware of whether the final product is going to be more dilute or more concentrated after the addition of more drug or diluent. When products are being formulated, it may be necessary to refer to official formulae and adapt the quantities, units of weight, volume or percentage to reflect the final amount to be prepared. There are numerous examples of this type of calculation included in this chapter. As in previous chapters, it is always important to standardise the units between the question and suggested answers at an early stage to minimise the errors that may occur.

After completing the questions in this chapter you should be able to:

- arrange pharmacopoeial formulae to prepare varying amounts of final product as units of weight, volume and percentages
- calculate the amount of active ingredient or diluent to alter the concentration of a solution or suspension
- express the concentration of a product in a number of ways, e.g. percentage strength and ratio
- use displacement values.

> **Directions for Questions 1–7.** In this section, each question or incomplete statement is followed by five suggested answers. Select the best answer in each case.

1 A manufacturer wishes to produce a batch of compressed tablets each containing 800 mg active ingredient, with a mean table weight of 1.2 g. Which of the following is the weight of active ingredient that will be required for a total batch size of 720 kg?

    A   600 kg
    B   400 kg
    C   250 kg
    D   480 kg
    E   420 kg

2 Your hospital pharmacy department has been asked to supply a 20 cm^2 bioadhesive patch containing 50 mg/cm^2 of 5-aminolevulinic hydrochloride (ALA) for use in a clinical trial on a named-patient basis. You know that 30 g aqueous gel containing ALA is required to prepare a patch of this drug loading 100 cm^2 in area. Which of the following is the concentration of ALA in an aqueous gel used to prepare the 20 cm^2 patch with an ALA loading of 50 mg/cm^2?

    A   1000 mg ALA in 6 g gel
    B   500 mg ALA in 6 g gel
    C   50 mg ALA in 20 g gel
    D   50 mg ALA in 30 g gel
    E   2000 mg ALA in 6 g gel

3 You have in your pharmacy an unopened 25 g tube of Metvix cream (16% w/w methylaminolevulinate). Which of the following is the amount of compatible diluent cream required to dilute this 25 g cream to a level of 4% methylaminolevulinate?

    A   25 g
    B   50 g
    C   75 g
    D   100 g
    E   125 g

4   An ointment has the following formula:
    Calamine 5%w/w
    Zinc oxide 10%w/w
    White Soft Paraffin, BP to 100%w/w
    Which of the following are the amounts of calamine and zinc oxide
    required to produce 80 g of this ointment?

    A   1.25 g calamine and 2.5 g zinc oxide
    B   2.5 g calamine and 5 g zinc oxide
    C   5 g calamine and 10 g zinc oxide
    D   8 g calamine and 16 g zinc oxide
    E   4 g calamine and 8 g zinc oxide

5   A patient has been prescribed 60 g of 0.2% w/w glyceryl trinitrate
    ointment for an anal fissure. The only strength glyceryl trinitrate
    ointment that you have available is 0.3% w/w. Which of the following
    is the amount of the 0.3% w/w glyceryl trinitrate ointment that you
    would need to prepare the required product?

    A   40 g
    B   50 g
    C   30 g
    D   20 g
    E   15 g

6   Which of the following is the volume of Molipaxin liquid (trazodone
    hydrochloride 50 mg/5 mL) required to be added to a suitable diluent
    to obtain 100 mL trazodone hydrochloride liquid 10 mg/5 mL?

    A   60 mL
    B   70 mL
    C   50 mL
    D   20 mL
    E   40 mL

7   Which of the following amounts of white soft paraffin is required to
    make 250 g of the product below?
    Zinc oxide 12% w/w
    Salicylic acid 1% w/w
    Starch 15% w/w
    White soft paraffin to 100% w/w

    A   70 g
    B   100 g

> C   150 g
> D   180 g
> E   200 g

Directions for Questions 8–10. For each numbered question, select the one lettered option that is most closely related to it. Within the group of questions, each lettered option may be used once, more than once or not at all.

Questions 8, 9 and 10 concern the following quantities:

> A   125 mg
> B   200 mg
> C   250 mg
> D   500 mg
> E   750 mg

Select, from A to E above, which is appropriate:

---

8   The amount of amoxicillin in a 5 mL dose if a bottle contains 2.5 g amoxicillin powder and the pharmacist adds 72 mL purified water to prepare 100 mL suspension.

9   The amount of betamethasone valerate in 200 g of a 0.1% w/w betamethasone valerate cream.

10   The amount of porfimer sodium in 20 mL of a 1 in 100 solution.

Directions for Questions 11 and 12. The questions in this section are followed by three responses. **ONE** or **MORE** of the responses is (are) correct. Decide which of the responses is (are) correct. Then choose:

Directions summarised:

A	B	C	D	E
1, 2, 3	1, 2 only	2, 3 only	1 only	3 only

---

11   The formula for Alkaline Gentian, Mixture, BP is:
Concentrated compound gentian infusion 100 mL

Sodium bicarbonate 50 g
Double-strength chloroform water 500 mL
Water to 1000 mL
Which of the following is/are correct?

1   The concentration of sodium bicarbonate in Alkaline Gentian, Mixture, BP is 5000 ppm
2   250 mL Alkaline Gentian, Mixture, BP contains 2.5 mL concentrated compound gentian infusion
3   10 mL Alkaline Gentian, Mixture, BP contains 5 mL double-strength chloroform water

12 The formula for 100 capsules is:
Paracetamol 50 g
Codeine phosphate 800 mg
Lactose 20 g
Which of the following is/are correct?

1   30 capsules contain 15 g paracetamol
2   A patient taking two capsules four times daily ingests 1.6 g lactose/day
3   15 capsules contain 120 mg codeine phosphate

Directions for Questions 13–19. In this section, each question or incomplete statement is followed by five suggested answers. Select the best answer in each case.

13 A vial containing 200 mg hydrocortisone sodium succinate powder for injection is to be reconstituted to produce 4 mL of injection. Which of the following is the amount of Water for Injections, BP that should be added to the powder? The displacement volume of hydrocortisone sodium succinate is 0.05 mL/100 mg.

A   2.0 mL
B   2.5 mL
C   3.5 mL
D   3.9 mL
E   4.0 mL

14 Which of the following is the volume of chlorhexidine gluconate 5% w/v solution that you would need to add to a suitable diluent to obtain 750 mL chlorhexidine gluconate 2% w/v solution?

A   75 mL
B   150 mL
C   250 mL
D   300 mL
E   500 mL

15 The formula for Chloral Elixir, Paediatric, BP is:
Chloral hydrate 200 mg
Water 0.1 mL
Blackcurrant syrup 1.0 mL
Syrup to 5.0 mL
You are presented with a prescription, for a 1-year-old child, for 150 mL Chloral Elixir, Paediatric, BP. You decide to make it up as an extemporaneous preparation. Which of the following is the amount of chloral hydrate that you would need?

A   0.3 g
B   3.0 g
C   6.0 g
D   0.6 g
E   10.0 g

16 You are requested to supply 250 g of a 1 in 4 dilution of Eumovate (0.05% w/w clobetasone butyrate) cream in aqueous cream. Which of the following are the correct amounts of the two creams that you would need?

A   112.5 g Eumovate plus 112.5 g aqueous cream
B   75 g Eumovate plus 175 g aqueous cream
C   50 g Eumovate plus 200 g aqueous cream
D   100 g Eumovate plus 150 g aqueous cream
E   62.5 g Eumovate plus 187.5 g aqueous cream

17 Which of the following is the percentage strength (w/w) of a saturated aqueous solution of sodium bicarbonate if it requires 20 mL water to just dissolve 2 g?

A   4.54%
B   9.09%
C   10%
D   10.9%
E   11.1%

18 Which of the following is the correct number of allopurinol 300 mg tablets required when preparing the following prescription for a gout patient who is currently unable to swallow tablets?
Allopurinol 50 mg/mL
Cherry syrup ad 150 mL
Signa (label) 10 mL in the morning after food

    A   20
    B   25
    C   10
    D   15
    E   40

19 Alupent syrup contains 10 mg/5 mL orciprenaline sulphate and Mucodyne oral liquid contains 125 mg/5 mL carbocisteine. Which of the following are the total daily doses of orciprenaline sulphate and carbocisteine received by a patient treated with 10 mL of the mixture below three times daily?
Alupent syrup/Mucodyne oral liquid 50/50 mix

    A   25 mg orciprenaline sulphate and 250 mg carbocisteine
    B   25 mg orciprenaline sulphate and 375 mg carbocisteine
    C   30 mg orciprenaline sulphate and 375 mg carbocisteine
    D   30 mg orciprenaline sulphate and 250 mg carbocisteine
    E   40 mg orciprenaline sulphate and 250 mg carbocisteine

Directions for Questions 20–22. For each numbered question, select the one lettered option that is most closely related to it. Within the group of questions, each lettered option may be used once, more than once or not at all.
Questions 20–22 concern the following quantities:

    A   24.5 mL
    B   4.85 mL
    C   19.85 mL
    D   15.45 mL
    E   3.65 mL

Select, from A to E above, which is appropriate:

20 The volume of Water for Injection, BP to be added to a vial containing 500 mg cyclophosphamide to produce 25 mL. The displacement volume of cyclophosphamide is 0.1 mL/100 mg.

21 The volume of Water for Injection, BP to be added to a vial containing 50 mg doxorubicin to produce an injection with a concentration of 2.5 mg/mL. The displacement volume of doxorubicin is 0.03 mL/10 mg.

22 The volume of water to be added to a vial containing 400 mg sodium valproate to produce a solution with a concentration of 100 mg/mL. The displacement volume of sodium valproate is 0.7 mL/800 mg.

Directions for Questions 23 and 24. The questions in this section are followed by three responses. ONE or MORE of the responses is (are) correct. Decide which of the responses is (are) correct. Then choose:

Directions summarised:

A	B	C	D	E
1, 2, 3	1, 2 only	2, 3 only	1 only	3 only

---

23 The formula for Paediatric Ferrous Sulphate Mixture is:
Ferrous sulphate 60 mg
Ascorbic acid 10 mg
Orange syrup 0.5 mL
Double-strength chloroform water 2.5 mL
Water to 5.0 mL
Which of the following is/are correct?

   1 The concentration of ascorbic acid in Paediatric Ferrous Sulphate Mixture is 20 mg/mL
   2 250 mL of Paediatric Ferrous Sulphate Mixture contains 25 mL orange syrup
   3 15 mL of Paediatric Ferrous Sulphate Mixture contains 7.5 mL double-strength chloroform water

24 The formula for coal tar and zinc ointment is:
Strong coal tar solution 100 g
Zinc oxide 300 g
Yellow soft paraffin 600 g
Which of the following is/are correct?

   1 The concentration of zinc oxide in coal tar and zinc ointment is 30% w/w

2 250 g coal tar and zinc ointment contains 25 g strong coal tar solution

3 The concentration of yellow soft paraffin in coal tar and zinc ointment is 50% w/w

Directions for Questions 25–31. In this section, each question or incomplete statement is followed by five suggested answers. Select the best answer in each case.

25 A manufacturer wishes to produce a batch of methylene blue gel for photodynamic antimicrobial chemotherapy of wound infections. The gel contains 20% w/w methylene blue. Which of the following is the weight of methylene blue that will be required for a total batch size of 360 kg?

    A   36 kg
    B   72 kg
    C   50 kg
    D   20 kg
    E   80 kg

26 Which of the following are the correct amounts of diclofenac sodium and misoprostol required to prepare 25 tablets according to the formula for an individual tablet given below?
Diclofenac sodium 50 mg
Misoprostol 200 micrograms
Lactose q.s. (sufficient quantity)

    A   1250 mg diclofenac sodium and 50 mg misoprostol
    B   1250 mg diclofenac sodium and 0.5 mg misoprostol
    C   250 mg diclofenac sodium and 5 mg misoprostol
    D   125 mg diclofenac sodium and 0.5 mg misoprostol
    E   1250 mg diclofenac sodium and 5 mg misoprostol

27 Which of the following is the amount of erythromycin ethyl succinate in 60 mL of a 500 mg/5 mL oral liquid?

    A   3 g
    B   12 g
    C   6 g
    D   60 g
    E   30 g

28 Which of the following is the amount of 20% w/w benzocaine ointment required to be added to a suitable diluent ointment to prepare 5 kg of a 2.5% w/w benzocaine ointment?

    A   2 kg
    B   6.25 g
    C   62. 5 g
    D   625.0 g
    E   2.5 kg

29 Which of the following is the number of furosemide 20 mg tablets required to prepare sufficient 50 mg/5 mL furosemide oral suspension to last 12 days for an infant taking 25 mg furosemide once daily?

    A   5
    B   10
    C   15
    D   20
    E   25

30 Your sterile manufacturing unit has been asked to supply eye drops with the following formula:
Dorzolamide hydrochloride 2% w/v
Timolol maleate 0.5% w/v
Which of the following are the correct amounts of the two drugs required to prepare 25 mL?

    A   5.000 mg dorzolamide hydrochloride and 0.125 mg timolol maleate
    B   500 mg dorzolamide hydrochloride and 12.5 mg timolol maleate
    C   125 mg dorzolamide hydrochloride and 500 mg timolol maleate
    D   12.5 mg dorzolamide hydrochloride and 500 mg timolol maleate
    E   500 mg dorzolamide hydrochloride and 125 mg timolol maleate

31 Which of the following is the concentration of glucose in a solution prepared by mixing 400 mL of 10% w/v glucose, 100 mL of 20% w/v glucose and 200 mL of 5% w/v glucose.

    A   5% w/v
    B   10% w/v
    C   12.5% w/v

D   15% w/v
E   17.5% w/v

Directions for Questions 32–34. For each numbered question, select the one lettered option that is most closely related to it. Within the group of questions, each lettered option may be used once, more than once or not at all.
Questions 32–34 concern the following quantities:

A   4 mL
B   16 mL
C   4.5 mL
D   2 mL
E   15 mL

Select, from A to E above, which is appropriate:

---

32   The amount of water required to dissolve 200 mg of a drug that has a solubility of 1 in 80 in water and 1 in 12 in alcohol.

33   The volume of glycerol required to prepare 15 mL of the following ear-drop formulation under sterile conditions:
Sodium bicarbonate 500 mg
Glycerol 3 mL
Water to 10 mL

34   The volume of phenoxymethylpenicillin suspension containing 100 mg drug if 5 g phenoxymethylpenicillin powder is made up to a final volume of 100 mL.

Directions for Questions 35 and 36. The questions in this section are followed by three responses. **ONE** or **MORE** of the responses is (are) correct. Decide which of the responses is (are) correct. Then choose:

Directions summarised:

A	B	C	D	E
1, 2, 3	1, 2 only	2, 3 only	1 only	3 only

35 The formula for Magnesium Trisilicate Mixture, BP is:
Magnesium trisilicate 50 g
Light magnesium carbonate 50 g
Sodium bicarbonate 50 g
Concentrated peppermint emulsion 25 mL
Double-strength chloroform water 500 mL water to 1000 mL
Which of the following is/are correct?

    1   The concentration of light magnesium carbonate in Magnesium Trisilicate Mixture, BP is 50 mg/mL

    2   500 mL Magnesium Trisilicate Mixture, BP contains 12.5 mL concentrated peppermint emulsion

    3   30 mL of Magnesium Trisilicate Mixture, BP contains 150 mg sodium bicarbonate

36 The formula for an extemporaneously prepared ointment is:
White soft paraffin 25 g
Betnovate ointment 20 g
Salicylic acid 5 g
Given that Betnovate ointment contains 0.1% w/w betamethasone valerate, which of the following is/are correct?

    1   The concentration of salicylic acid in this extemporaneously prepared ointment is 5% w/w

    2   The concentration of betamethasone valerate in this extemporaneously prepared ointment is 0.02% w/w

    3   75 g of white soft paraffin would be required to prepare 150 g of this extemporaneously prepared ointment

Directions for Questions 37–43. In this section, each question or incomplete statement is followed by five suggested answers. Select the best answer in each case.

Questions 37 and 38. During the manufacture of suppositories, there is a calculation step that has no direct equivalent in the manufacture of other products. A drug will displace a certain amount of suppository base, depending on its density. This amount is given by its 'displacement value'. A displacement value (DV) of 2 means that 2 g of the drug will displace 1 g of the suppository base. As suppository moulds are filled by volume not weight, the DV values of the drug are taken into account when formulating the product. The amount of suppository base required can be calculated knowing the amount of base required if no drug was to be incorporated and the DV value of the drug to be incorporated in the suppositories, as follows:

Amount of base required = theoretical amount – displaced amount = theoretical amount – (amount of drug in g/DV of drug).

Pessaries are formulated on exactly the same principles as suppositories.

37 You are asked to prepare and dispense 6 × 1 g suppositories, each containing 150 mg bismuth subnitrate. Allowing for a 50% excess (i.e. calculating on the basis that a total of nine suppositories will be prepared), which of the following are the amounts of suppository base and bismuth subnitrate required for correct formulation of these suppositories? The displacement value of bismuth subnitrate is 5.

    A 0.9 g bismuth subnitrate and 6.0 g suppository base
    B 1.35 g bismuth subnitrate and 9.00 g suppository base
    C 1.35 g bismuth subnitrate and 8.73 g suppository base
    D 1 g bismuth subnitrate and 8 g suppository base
    E 8 g bismuth subnitrate and 1 g suppository base

38 You are asked to prepare and dispense six 4 g vaginal pessaries, each containing 500 mg clotrimazole. Allowing for a 50% excess (i.e. calculating on the basis that a total of nine pessaries will be prepared), which of the following are the amounts of suppository base and clotrimazole that will be required for correct formulation of these pessaries? The displacement value of clotrimazole is 1.5.

    A 0.5 g clotrimazole and 6.0 g pessary base
    B 4.5 g clotrimazole and 24 g pessary base
    C 3 g clotrimazole and 33 g pessary base
    D 3 g clotrimazole and 24 g pessary base
    E 4.5 g clotrimazole and 33 g pessary base

39 Which of the following is the correct number of spironolactone 25 mg tablets required to prepare 200 mL of a paediatric oral suspension containing 5 mg/mL spironolactone?

    A 40
    B 20
    C 30

> **D** 10
> **E** 50

40 A rectal gel is prepared according to the formulation below:
Lorazepam 80 mg
Methylcellulose 2.5 g
Methylparaben 100 mg
Glycerol 5 g
Water to 100 mL
Which of the following is the number of 1 mL ampoules of Ativan injection (lorazepam 4 mg/mL) required to prepare 25 g of this gel correctly?

> **A** 2
> **B** 3
> **C** 4
> **D** 5
> **E** 6

41 Which of the following is the volume of Water for Injection, BP to be added to a vial containing 500 mg amoxicillin to produce a solution with a volume of 5 mL. The displacement volume of amoxicillin is 0.1 mL for 125 mg.

> **A** 4.6 mL
> **B** 3.0 mL
> **C** 3.6 mL
> **D** 5.0 mL
> **E** 4.5 mL

42 Which of the following is the amount of codeine hydrochloride (solubility 1 in 20 of water) that will dissolve in 150 mL water?

> **A** 15.5 g
> **B** 8.5 g
> **C** 7.5 g
> **D** 5.5 g
> **E** 4.5 g

43 Ergometrine maleate has a solubility of 1 in 40 in water. Which of the following is the amount of water required to dissolve 2.5 g ergometrine maleate?

> **A** 25 mL
> **B** 80 mL

C   50 mL
D   100 mL
E   125 mL

Directions for Questions 44–46. For each numbered question, select the one lettered option that is most closely related to it. Within the group of questions, each lettered option may be used once, more than once or not at all.

Questions 44–46 concern the following quantities:

A   4.0 g
B   10.0 g
C   2.5 g
D   9.0 g
E   15.3 g

Select, from A to E above, which is appropriate:

44   The amount of suppository base required (allowing for a 50% excess, i.e. calculating on the basis that a total of nine suppositories will be prepared) in the correct formulation of six 2 g suppositories each containing 0.3 mL belladonna tincture. Belladonna tincture has a displacement value of 1. It is known that, in the formulation of suppositories:
Amount of base required = theoretical amount − (amount of drug in g/DV of drug).

45   The amount of captopril contained in 2.5 L of a suspension made according to the following formulation:
Captopril 100 mg tablet
Keltrol suspension 50 mL
Water to 100 mL

46   The amount of hydrocortisone cream 1% w/w required to be added to a suitable diluent cream to prepare 20 g of a 0.5% w/w hydrocortisone cream.

Directions for Questions 47 and 48. The questions in this section are followed by three responses. **ONE** or **MORE** of the responses is (are) correct. Decide which of the responses is (are) correct. Then choose:

Directions summarised:

A	B	C	D	E
1, 2, 3	1, 2 only	2, 3 only	1 only	3 only

47 The formula for Ammonia and Ipecacuanha Mixture, BP is:

Ammonium bicarbonate 200 mg
Liquorice liquid extract 0.5 mL
Ipecacuanha tincture 0.3 mL
Concentrated camphor water 0.1 mL
Concentrated anise water 0.05 mL
Double-strength chloroform water 5 mL
Water to 10 mL
Which of the following is/are correct?

  1 The concentration of ammonium bicarbonate in Ammonia and
     Ipecacuanha Mixture, BP is 2 mg/mL
  2 500 mL of Ammonia and Ipecacuanha Mixture, BP contains
     5 mL concentrated camphor water
  3 30 mL of Ammonia and Ipecacuanha Mixture, BP contains 15
     mL double-strength chloroform water

48 You are asked to prepare six 1 g suppositories, each containing 100 mg
   bismuth subnitrate and 200 mg paracetamol. The displacement value
   of bismuth subnitrate is 5.0 and of paracetamol is 1.5. It is known that,
   in the formulation of suppositories:
   Amount of base required = theoretical amount − (amount of drug in
   g/DV of drug).
   Allowing for a 50% excess (i.e. calculating on the basis that a total of
   nine suppositories will be prepared) which of the following is/are
   correct?

  1 The amount of suppository base required is 7.62 g
  2 The amount of paracetamol required is 1.8 g
  3 The amount of bismuth subnitrate required is 0.9 g

Directions for Questions 49–55. In this section, each question or incomplete statement is followed by five suggested answers. Select the best answer in each case.

49 Which of the following is the amount of Codeine Linctus, BP (codeine phosphate 15 mg/5 mL) required to be added to a suitable diluent to prepare 75 mL Codeine Linctus, Paediatric, BP (codeine phosphate 3 mg/5 mL)?

    A   20 mL
    B   15 mL
    C   10 mL
    D   25 mL
    E   45 mL

50 The formula for a single capsule filled extemporaneously for use in a clinical trial is:
Estriol 250 micrograms
Estradiol 190 micrograms
Starch 320 mg
Which of the following is the amount of estriol required to produce 50 tablets?

    A   12.50 mg
    B   1.25 mg
    C   125.00 mg
    D   250.00 mg
    E   25.00 mg

51 Which of the following are the correct amounts of 50 mg/5 mL and 200 mg/5 mL phenytoin sodium suspensions required to prepare 200 mL of an 80 mg/5 mL suspension?

    A   80 mL of the 200 mg/5 mL suspension and 120 mL of the 50 mg/5 mL suspension
    B   50 mL of the 200 mg/5 mL suspension and 150 mL of the 50 mg/5 mL suspension
    C   100 mL of the 200 mg/5 mL suspension and 100 mL of the 50 mg/5 mL suspension
    D   40 mL of the 200 mg/5 mL suspension and 160 mL of the 50 mg/5 mL suspension
    E   160 mL of the 200 mg/5 mL suspension and 40 mL of the 50 mg/5 mL suspension

52 Which of the following are the correct amounts (to one decimal place) of clotrimazole 1% w/w cream and clotrimazole powder required to produce 75 g of 3% w/w clotrimazole cream?

A   1.5 g of the powder and 73.5 g of the 1% w/w cream
B   73.5 g of the powder and 1.5 g of the 1% w/w cream
C   25 g of the powder and 75 g of the 1% w/w cream
D   75 g of the powder and 25 g of the 1% w/w cream
E   37.5 g of the powder and 37.5 g of the 1% w/w cream

53 The formula for a single powder for oral use is given as:
Aspirin 600 mg
Aloxiprin 150 mg
Caffeine 250 mg
Which of the following is the concentration of caffeine in this powder?

A   25.0% w/w
B   12.5% w/w
C   15.0% w/w
D   10.0% w/w
E   20.0% w/w

54 Which of the following is the volume of a 4 mg/mL suspension of drug G that you would prepare for a patient who required 14 mg twice daily for 7 days?

A   14 mL
B   28 mL
C   50 mL
D   49 mL
E   15 mL

55 You add 90 mL of 4.5% w/v sodium chloride solution to a 500 mL infusion bag of 0.9%w/v sodium chloride solution to obtain the correct level of NaCl for infusion to a patient. Which of the following is the final concentration of the solution? Assume no volume displacement effects.

A   1.45% w/v
B   14.50% w/v
C   4.50% w/v
D   4.00% w/v
E   1.00% w/v

Directions for Questions 56–58. For each numbered question, select the one lettered option that is most closely related to it. Within the group of questions, each lettered option may be used once, more than once or not at all.

Questions 56–58 concern the following quantities:

    A   1.0 g
    B   10.0 g
    C   3.0 g
    D   2.5 g
    E   1.25 g

Select, from A to E above, which is appropriate:

56 The amount of toluidine blue O required to prepare a $25 \, cm^2$ mucoadhesive patch for photodynamic therapy of oral candidiasis if the desired drug loading is $50 \, mg/cm^2$.

57 The amount of hexylaminolevulinate contained in 75 mL of a 4.0% w/w solution for instillation into the bladder for photodynamic diagnosis of bladder cancer.

58 The amount of ketoconazole in 100 g of a cream prepared according to the following formula:
Nizoral cream 50%
Aqueous cream 50%
Nizoral cream containing 2.0% w/w ketoconazole.

Directions for Questions 59 and 60. The questions in this section are followed by three responses. **ONE** or **MORE** of the responses is (are) correct. Decide which of the responses is (are) correct. Then choose:

Directions summarised:				
A	B	C	D	E
1, 2, 3	1, 2 only	2, 3 only	1 only	3 only

59 You receive a prescription to prepare 500 mL of a mixture composed of:

Motilium suspension 1 part

Kolanticon gel 2 parts

Zantac syrup 2 parts

Given that Motilium suspension contains 5 mg/5 mL of domperidone, Kolanticon gel contains 2.5 mg/5 mL of dicycloverine hydrochloride and Zantac syrup contains 75 mg/5 mL of ranitidine hydrochloride, which of the following is/are correct?

    1   100 mL of the mixture contains 20 mg domperidone

    2   100 mL of the mixture contains 20 mg dicycloverine hydrochloride

    3   100 mL of the mixture contains 20 mg ranitidine hydrochloride

60 You are asked to prepare the following ear-drop formulation under aseptic conditions:

Hydrogen peroxide solution (6% v/v) 25%

Water 75%

Which of the following is/are correct?

    1   100 mL of the ear-drop formulation contains 25 mL hydrogen peroxide

    2   40 mL of the ear-drop formulation contains 35 mL water

    3   50 mL of the ear-drop formulation contains 12.5 mL hydrogen peroxide solution

ANSWERS

1 D
Every 1200 mg tablet contains 800 mg active drug, so 800/1200 = 2/3 of each tablet is drug
Accordingly, two-thirds of the batch size of 720 kg must be drug.
720/3 = 240
240 × 2 = 480 kg.
Therefore, the correct answer is D.

2 A
If the drug loading is 50 mg/cm^2 and the patch area is 20 cm^2, then 1000 mg ALA are required
If 30 g gel is required to make a patch 100 cm^2 in area, then 6 g gel are required for a 20 cm^2 patch.
Therefore, the correct answer is A.

3 C
Dilution factor = (initial concn)/(final concn) = (16% w/w)/(4% w/w) = 4
Therefore, the original cream needs to be diluted 1 in 4, i.e. 1 part original cream and 3 parts diluent cream
Quantity of diluent cream required = 3 × 25 g = 75 g.
Accordingly, the correct answer is C.

4 E
This question can be answered by simple multiplication and division as follows:
(80/100) × 10 = 8
10% of 80 g is, therefore, 8 g
(80/100) × 5 = 4
so 5% of 80 g is 4 g
The correct answer is E.

5 A
60 g of a 0.2% w/w ointment contains: (60/100) × 0.2 = 0.12 g glyceryl trinitrate
The 0.3% w/w ointment contains 0.3 g glyceryl trinitrate in 100 g, or 0.03 g in 10 g
0.03 g × 4 = 0.12 g

Accordingly, 40 g of the 0.3% w/w ointment will be required.
The correct answer is, therefore, A.

6 D
100 mL of a 10 mg/5 mL syrup contains 200 mg trazodone hydrochloride
Molipaxin liquid contains 50 mg/5 mL of trazodone hydrochloride
200 mg/50 mg = 4
Hence, 4 × 5 mL aliquots are required = 20 mL.
The correct answer is D.

7 D
First, add up all the other ingredients. This comes to 28%. Therefore, white soft paraffin must constitute 72% of the final product.
250/100 × 72 = 180 g.
Accordingly, the correct answer is D.

8 A
There are 2.5 g, or 2500 mg in 100 mL of suspension, so there must be 25 mg in 1 mL and 125 mg in 5 mL.
The correct answer is A.

9 B
This is a case of simple multiplication and division, as follows:
(200/100) × 0.1 = 0.2 g, or 200 mg.
Accordingly, the correct answer is B.

10 B
In a 1 in 100 solution, there is 1 g or 1000 mg in 100 mL; 20 mL must, therefore, contain 200 mg.
Therefore, the correct answer is B.

11 E
1   A 1 ppm solution contains 1 g in 1000 000 mL; Alkaline Gentian, Mixture, BP contains 50 g sodium bicarbonate in 1000 mL, or 50 000 g in 1000 000 mL. Therefore, the sodium bicarbonate is 50 000 ppm.
2   1000 mL of Alkaline Gentian, Mixture, BP contains 100 mL concentrated compound gentian infusion, so dividing both by 4 gives 25 mL concentrated compound gentian infusion in 250 mL Alkaline Gentian Mixture.

3 1000 mL Alkaline Gentian, Mixture, BP contains 500 mL, so 10 mL must contain 5 mL.
Accordingly, only 3 is true, so the correct answer is E.

12 A

1 If 50 g paracetamol are required for 100 capsules, each capsule must contain 0.5 g or 500 mg. Accordingly, 30 capsules contain 15 g paracetamol.
2 The patient takes 8 capsules/day; 100 capsules contain 20 g lactose: $(20/100) \times 8 = 1.6$ g lactose.
3 If 800 mg codeine phosphate are required for 100 capsules, each capsule must contain 8 mg: $15 \times 8 = 120$ mg codeine phosphate.
All three statements are true, so the correct answer is A.

13 D

The displacement volume indicates that 100 mg hydrocortisone sodium succinate will occupy the volumeof 0.05 mL water
Therefore, 200 mg will occupy the volume of 0.1 mL water
Accordingly, the volume of Water for Injection, BP to be added is 4 mL – 0.1 mL = 3.9 mL.
The correct answer is D.

14 D

100 mL of a 2% w/v solution contains 2 g chlorhexidine gluconate
750 mL must contain 15 g
100 mL of a 5% w/v solution contains 5 g chlorhexidine gluconate
Therefore, 15 g must be contained in 300 mL.
The correct answer is D.

15 C

There are 200 mg of chloral hydrate in every 5.0 mL, so in 150 mL there must be:
200 mg × 30 = 6000 mg, or 6.0 g.
The correct answer is C.

16 E

The concentration of clobetasone butyrate in the cream is irrelevant here. First, split 250 g into four parts, each of 62.5 g. One part (62.5 g) will be Eumovate and the other three parts (187.5 g) will be aqueous cream. Therefore, the correct answer is E.

17 B
2 g added to 20 mL water gives a solution of 22 g, as 1 mL water weighs 1 g
$(2/22) \times 100 = 9.09\%$ w/w.
The correct answer is B.

18 B
Each 1 mL of the suspension contains 50 mg allopurinol
In 150 mL there is:
50 mg $\times$ 150 = 7500 mg
Each tablet contains 300 mg, so:
7500/300 = 25 tablets required.
The correct answer is B.

19 C
If we consider Alupent and Mucodyne as though they were separate dosage forms, the patient receives 5 mL of each three times daily
Alupent syrup contains 10 mg/5 mL orciprenaline sulphate, so the patient gets 30 mg orciprenaline sulphate/day
Mucodyne oral liquid contains 125 mg/5 mL carbocisteine so the patient gets 375 mg carbocisteine/day.
Accordingly, the correct answer is C.

20 A
100 mg cyclophosphamide displace 0.1 mL, so 500 mg must displace 0.5 mL
Accordingly, 24.5 mL Water for Injection, BP must be added.
The correct answer is therefore A.

21 C
A 2.5 mg/mL solution contains 2.5 mg in 1 mL, or 50 mg in 20 mL
The final volume required must be 20 mL
10 mg doxorubicin displace 0.03 mL, so 50 mg must displace 0.15 mL
20 mL – 0.15 mL = 19.85 mL Water for Injection, BP must be added.
The correct answer is therefore C.

22 E
A 100 mg/mL solution contains 100 mg in 1 mL, or 400 mg in 4 mL
The final volume required must be 4 mL

800 mg sodium valproate displace 0.7 mL, so 400 mg must displace 0.35 mL
4 mL – 0.35 mL = 3.65 mL water must be added.
The correct answer is therefore E.

23 C
1   There are 10 mg ascorbic acid in 5.0 mL Paediatric Ferrous Sulphate Mixture, so there must be 2 mg in 1 mL. The concentration is 2 mg/mL.
2   5 mL of Paediatric Ferrous Sulphate Mixture contains 0.5 mL orange syrup, so multiplying both by 50 gives 25 mL orange syrup in 250 mL Paediatric Ferrous Sulphate Mixture.
3   5 mL of Paediatric Ferrous Sulphate Mixture contains 2.5 mL double-strength chloroform water, so 15 mL must contain 7.5 mL.
Accordingly, 2 and 3 are true, so the correct answer is C.

24 B
1   First add up the amounts of all the ingredients. This comes to 1000 g. In 1000 g we have 300 g zinc oxide
    $300/1000 \times 100 = 30\%$ w/w.
2   In 1000 g of 5 mL coal tar and zinc ointment we have 100 g strong coal tar solution. Dividing both by 4 gives us 25 g in 250 g.
3   In 1000 g we have 600 g yellow soft paraffin
    $600/1000 \times 100 = 60\%$ w/w.
Accordingly, 1 and 2 are true, so the correct answer is B.

25 B
Every 100 kg of gel contains 20 kg methylene blue, so $(20/100) \times 360 = 72$ kg.
Therefore, the correct answer is B.

26 E
This is simply a case of multiplication, as follows:
Diclofenac sodium: $50 \text{ mg} \times 25 = 1250$ mg
Misoprostol: 200 micrograms $= 0.2$ mg; $0.2 \text{ mg} \times 25 = 5$ mg.
Accordingly, the correct answer is E.

27 C
The liquid contains 500 mg in 5 mL
Multiplying by 12 gives the amount in 60 mL, which is 6000 mg or 6 g.
The correct answer is C.

28 D
A 2.5% w/w ointment contains 2.5 g benzocaine in 100 g or 25 g benzocaine in 1000 g or 1 kg
There must be 5×25 g = 125 g benzocaine in 5 kg
A 20% w/w ointment contains 20 g benzocaine in 100 g
125/20 = 6.25
6.25×100 = 625 g of 20% w/w ointment required.
The correct answer is D.

29 C
First calculate the total amount of furosemide required.
The dose is 25 mg daily for 12 days
This equates with 300 mg
300/20 = 15 tablets required
As the oral suspension has a concentration of 50 mg/5 mL and we must deliver 300 mg, these tablets would need to be crushed to a uniform powder and suspended appropriately to give a final volume of 30 mL.
The correct answer is C.

30 E
Consider each drug in turn:
Dorzolamide hydrochloride: 2% w/v = 2 g in 100 mL or 0.5 g in 25 mL; this equates with 500 mg
Timolol maleate: 0.5% w/v = 0.5 g in 100 mL or 0.125 g in 25 mL; this equates with 125 mg.
The correct answer is E.

31 B
First add up all the volumes: 400 mL + 100 mL + 200 mL = 700 mL
Now work out the total amount of glucose:
400 mL of a 10% w/v solution contains 40 g
100 mL of a 20% w/v solution contains 20 g
200 mL of a 5% w/v solution contains 10 g
Adding these amounts we have: 40 g + 20 g + 10 g = 70 g
In the final solution we have 70 g in 700 mL; this equates to 10 g in 100 mL, so we have a 10% w/v solution of glucose.
The correct answer is B.

32 B
1 g, or 1000 mg, of the drug will dissolve in 80 mL water

Divide both by 5 and we find that 1000 mg/5 = 200 mg
80 mL/5 = 16 mL.
The correct answer is B.

33 C
This is a case of simple multiplication
If 3 mL glycerol is required for 10 mL ear drops, then 4.5 mL is required for 15 mL.
Accordingly, the correct answer is C.

34 E
If we have 5 g in 100 mL, this means that we have 5000 mg in 100 mL, or 50 mg in 1 mL
100 mg will be contained in 2 mL of the final suspension.
The correct answer is E.

35 B
1   There are 50 g, or 50 000 mg light magnesium carbonate in 1000 mL Magnesium Trisilicate Mixture, BP, so there must be 50 mg in 1 mL. The concentration is 50 mg/mL.
2   1000 mL Magnesium Trisilicate Mixture, BP contains 25 mL concentrated peppermint emulsion, so dividing both by 2 gives 12.5 mL concentrated peppermint emulsion in 500 mL Magnesium Trisilicate Mixture, BP.
3   1000 mL Magnesium Trisilicate Mixture, BP contains 50 g sodium bicarbonate, or 50 000 mg, so there must be 50 mg in 1 mL and 50 × 30 =1500 mg in 30 mL.
Accordingly, 1 and 2 are true and so the correct answer is B.

36 E
1   In 50 g of the ointment we have 5 g salicylic acid, so in 100 g we would have 10 g. Accordingly the concentration of salicylic acid is 10% w/w.
2   100 g Betnovate ointment contains 0.1 g betamethasone valerate, so 20 g contains 0.1 g/5 = 0.02 g. The final weight of ointment, containing 20 g Betnovate ointment, is 50 g, so we have 0.02 g in 50 g or 0.04 g in 100 g. The betamethasone valerate concentration is 0.04% w/w.
3   In 50 g of ointment we have 25 g white soft paraffin, so multiplying by 3 gives us 75 g in 150 g.
As 3 only is true, the correct answer is E.

37 C
A displacement value (DV) of 5 means that 5 g of the drug will displace 1 g suppository base
Bismuth subnitrate has a DV of 5, i.e. 5 g bismuth subnitrate displaces 1 g suppository base
Amount of base required = theoretical amount − displaced amount
(Calculating for nine suppositories) = (9 × 1 g) − (amount of drug/DV of drug)
= (9 × 1 g) − (1.35 g/5)
= 9 g − 0.27 g
= 8.73 g
Final formulation is: bismuth subnitrate 1.35 g, suppository base 8.73 g.
The correct answer is C.

38 E
A displacement value (DV) of 1.5 means that 1.5 g of the drug will displace 1 g pessary base
Clotrimazole has a DV of 1.5, i.e. 1.5 g clotrimazole displaces 1 g suppository base
Amount of base required = theoretical amount − displaced amount
= (9 × 4 g) − (amount of drug/DV of drug)
= (9 × 4 g) − (4.5 g/1.5)
= 36.0 g − 3.0 g
= 33.0 g
Final formulation is: clotrimazole 4.5 g, pessary base 33.0 g.
The correct answer is E.

39 A
200 mL of a 5 mg/mL suspension contains 5 × 200 = 1000 mg spironolactone
1000/25 = 40 tablets required.
The correct answer is A.

40 D
If there are 80 mg lorazepam in 100 mL gel, there must be 20 mg in 25 mL
Each vial of Ativan contains 4 mg lorazepam, so five vials are required.
The correct answer is D.

41 A
125 mg amoxicillin displace 0.1 mL, so 500 mg must displace 0.4 mL

5 mL – 0.4 mL = 4.6 mL water must be added.
The correct answer is A.

42 C
This is a case of simple multiplication and division:
1 g will dissolve in 20 mL
150 mL/20 = 7.5 g will dissolve in 150 mL.
The correct answer is C.

43 D
This is, again, a case of simple multiplication and division:
1 g will dissolve in 40 mL
Multiplying by 2.5 tells us that 2.5 g will dissolve in 100 mL
The correct answer is D.

44 E
As it is a liquid, belladonna tincture has a displacement value (DV) of 1,
i.e. 1 mL belladonna tincture displaces 1 g suppository base
Amount of base required = theoretical amount – displaced amount
= (9 × 2 g) – (amount of drug/DV of drug)
= (9 × 2 g) – (2.7/1)
= 18 g – 2.7 g
= 15.3 g
Final formulation is Belladonna Tincture, BP 2.7 mL, suppository base
15.3 g.
The correct answer is E.

45 C
100 mL contains 100 mg, so 2500 mL must contain 2500 mg, or 2.5 g.
The correct answer is C.

46 B
If the concentration of the new cream is 0.5% w/w, we have done a 1 in 2
dilution, i.e. the original cream is 50% of the new cream and so we need
10 g of the original cream.
The correct answer is B.

47 C
1   There are 200 mg ammonium bicarbonate in 10 mL Ammonia and
    Ipecacuanha Mixture, BP, so there must be 20 mg in 1 mL and its
    concentration is 20 mg/mL.

2   10 mL of Ammonia and Ipecacuanha Mixture, BP contains 0.1 mL concentrated camphor water, so 500 mL contains $50 \times 0.1 = 5$ mL.

3   10 mL Ammonia and Ipecacuanha Mixture, BP contains 5 mL double-strength chloroform water, so 30 mL contains $3 \times 5 = 15$ mL.

As 2 and 3 only are true, the correct answer is C.

48 A

Amount of base required = theoretical amount – displaced amount (bismuth subnitrate) – displaced amount (paracetamol)

= $(9 \times 1 \text{ g}) - ([\text{amount of drug/DV}]$ for bismuth subnitrate) $- ([\text{amount of drug/DV}]$ for paracetamol)

= $(9 \times 1 \text{ g}) - (0.9 \text{ g/5}) - (1.8/1.5)$

= $9 \text{ g} - 0.18 \text{ g} - 1.2 \text{ g}$

= 7.62 g

Final formulation is bismuth subnitrate 0.9 g, paracetamol 1.8 g, suppository base 7.62 g

Accordingly, 1, 2 and 3 above are true and so the correct answer is A.

49 B

Codeine Linctus, Paediatric, BP contains 3 mg codeine phosphate in 5 mL, so it contains 45 mg in 75 mL

Codeine Linctus, BP contains 15 mg codeine phosphate in 5 mL

Therefore, 15 mL are required for 45 mL.

The correct answer is B.

50 A

This is a case of simple multiplication:

250 micrograms is equivalent to 0.25 mg

$0.25 \text{ g} \times 50 = 12.5$ mg.

The correct answer is A.

51 D

This question requires use of alligation alternate.

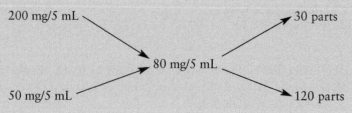

Total number of parts = 30 parts + 120 parts = 150 parts, which is equivalent to 200 mL. We can thus use simple proportion to calculate:
Amount of 200 mg/5 mL phenytoin sodium suspension = (30 × 200)/150 = 40 mL
Amount of 50 mg/5 mL phenytoin sodium suspension = (120 × 200)/150 = 160 mL.
The correct answer is D.

52 D
This question requires use of alligation alternate.

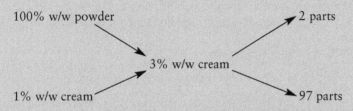

Total number of parts = 2 parts + 97 parts = 99 parts, which is equivalent to 75 g. We can thus use simple proportion to calculate:
Amount of 100% w/w powder = (2 × 75)/99 = 1.5 g
Amount of 1% w/w cream = (97 × 75)/99 = 73.5 g.
The correct answer is D.

53 A
The ingredients add up to 1000 mg, of which 250 mg is caffeine, so the caffeine concentration must be 25% w/w.
The correct answer is A.

54 D
We require 14 mg per dose, supplied as 4 mg/mL
Volume per dose = (14 mg)/(4 mg/mL) = 3.5 mL
Total volume required = volume per dose × frequency × duration
= 3.5 mL × 2 × 7 = 49 mL.
The correct answer is D.

55 A
Final solution = 90 mL 4.5% sodium chloride solution + 500 mL 0.9%w/v sodium chloride solution = 590 mL
Sodium chloride from each solution:

0.9% w/v sodium chloride = 0.9 g in 100 mL = (0.9 × 500)/100 = 4.5 g sodium chloride in 500 mL
4.5% w/v sodium chloride = 4.5 g in 100 mL = (4.5 × 90)/100 = 4.05 g sodium chloride in 90 mL
Total sodium chloride = 4.5 + 4.05 = 8.55 g
Therefore, the final concentration = 8.55 g in 590 mL = 1.45 g in 100 mL = 1.45% w/v.
The correct answer is, therefore, A.

56 E
If 50 mg is required for each square centimetre:
25 × 50 = 1250 mg, or 1.25 g toluidine blue O, is required for a 25 cm^2 patch.
Accordingly, the correct answer is E.

57 C
In 100 mL of a 4.0% w/w solution, there are 4.0 g hexylaminolevulinate
In 75 mL there must be: (4/100) × 75 = 3.0 g.
The correct answer is C.

58 A
The final cream will contain 50 g Nizoral cream
As Nizoral cream is 2.0% w/w ketoconazole, and has been diluted 1 in 2, the final cream will contain 1.0 g in 100 g.
Accordingly, the correct answer is A.

59 B
Consider 100 mL in parts, as outlined in the formula. There are 5 × 20 mL parts, so:
Motilium suspension 20 mL
Kolanticon gel 40 mL
Zantac syrup 40 mL
1   Motilium suspension contains 5 mg/5 mL of domperidone, so, in 20 mL, there will be 20 mg domperidone.
2   Kolanticon gel contains 2.5 mg/5 mL of dicycloverine hydrochloride, so, in 40 mL, there will be 20 mg dicycloverine hydrochloride.
3   Zantac syrup contains 75 mg/5 mL of ranitidine hydrochloride, so, in 40 mL, there will be 600 mg ranitidine hydrochloride.
As only 1 and 2 are true, the correct answer is B.

60 E

1 100 mL of the ear-drop formulation contains 25 mL hydrogen peroxide solution. However, this solution is only 6% v/v hydrogen peroxide. The amount of hydrogen peroxide in 25 mL is $(25/100) \times 6 = 1.5$ mL.

2 As the ear-drop formulation is 75% water, the amount of water in 40 mL is:

$(40/100) \times 75 = 30$ mL.

3 The ear-drop formulation is 25% hydrogen peroxide solution, so $50/100 \times 25 = 12.5$ mL hydrogen peroxide solution.

Therefore, only 3 is true, so the correct answer is E.

5 Pharmaceutical chemistry

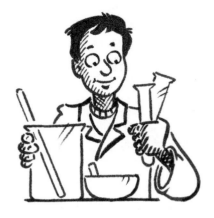

Chemistry is the science that underpins the profession of pharmacy. Chemistry-related calculations differ significantly from those used in other areas of pharmaceutical practice. However, these types of calculations are routinely carried out by pharmacy students over the course of their undergraduate programme and also by pharmacists working within the pharmaceutical sciences in academia or industry. The questions in this chapter help the reader gain experience in calculations related to the differing chemical forms of the active ingredient in formulated products, chemical synthesis of drugs, drug degradation processes and pharmaceutical analysis.

After completing the questions in this chapter you should be able to:

- calculate the amount of parent drug in a dosage form containing a drug salt or other derivative
- predict the shelf-lives of pharmaceutical products
- determine drug concentration using analytical data
- identify products not complying with the appropriate pharmacopoeial monograph.

QUESTIONS

Directions for Questions 1–7. In this section, each question or incomplete statement is followed by five suggested answers. Select the best answer in each case.

1 The manufacturer of ferrous gluconate cannot supply due to a fire in the main manufacturing plant. Your patient normally takes two tablets once daily. They are now being given Plesmet syrup as an alternative. They need to receive exactly the same amount of iron. Which of the following would be an appropriate dose of this syrup? Ferrous gluconate tablets contain 35 mg iron per tablet. Plesmet syrup contains 25 mg iron/5 mL.

    A   5 mL three times daily
    B   6 mL twice daily
    C   7 mL once daily
    D   7 mL twice daily
    E   5 mL once daily

2 How much active substance is required to manufacture a batch of granules for a compressed tablet with a batch size of 420 kg, to produce tablets with a mean weight of 700 mg and an active substance content of 600 mg?

    A   400 kg
    B   380 kg
    C   378 kg
    D   360 kg
    E   265 kg

3 Given that the relative molecular mass (RMM) of sodium chloride is 58.5 g/mol, which of the following amounts of sodium chloride powder would be required to prepare 300 mL of a solution containing 50 mmol/L?

    A   0.878 g
    B   0.585 g
    C   1.75 g
    D   1.14 g
    E   1.5 g

4   A tablet labelled to contain 350 mg active ingredient has acceptable limits of 90–110% of that amount. Which of the following indicates the limits of content?

    A   300–400 mg
    B   310–390 mg
    C   315–385 mg
    D   320–380 mg
    E   340–360 mg

5   Ranitidine tablets are available as tablets containing ranitidine hydrochloride equivalent to 150 mg and 300 mg ranitidine. For ranitidine 150 mg tablets, which of the following amounts of ranitidine hydrochloride is needed in each tablet? (RMM: ranitidine, $C_{13}H_{22}N_4O_3S$ = 314.4 g/mol; ranitidine hydrochloride, $C_{13}H_{22}N_4O_3S.HCl$ = 350.9 g/mol.)

    A   134.55 mg
    B   167.41 mg
    C   172.35 mg
    D   122.98 mg
    E   150.00 mg

6   Which of the following amounts of sodium ions does 50 mL sodium chloride solution 0.9% w/v intravenous infusion contain? There are 150 mmol each of Na^+ and Cl^-/L of NaCl 0.9% w/v IV infusion.

    A   0.0075 mmol
    B   0.075 mmol
    C   7.5 mmol
    D   15 mmol
    E   0.15 mmol

7   Ferrous gluconate tablets are out of stock and your patient normally takes two tablets once daily. The GP has prescribed Galfer syrup as an alternative. The patient needs to receive the same amount of iron. Which of the following would be an appropriate dose of Galfer syrup? Ferrous gluconate contains 35 mg iron. Galfer syrup contains 45 mg iron/5 mL.

    A   15.6 mL twice daily
    B   7.8 mL once daily
    C   7.8 mL twice daily
    D   15.6 mL once daily
    E   15.6 mL three times daily

Directions for Questions 8–10 For each numbered question, select the one lettered option that is most closely related to it. Within the group of questions, each lettered option may be used once, more than once or not at all.

Questions 8–10 concern the following quantities:

    A   2.040 g
    B   2.500 g
    C   2.925 g
    D   2.870 g
    E   2.245 g

Select, from A to E above, which is appropriate:

8   The amount of sodium chloride required to make 500 mL of a 0.1 mol/L solution (relative atomic mass [RAM]: sodium = 23; chlorine = 35.5.)

9   The amount of lymeycline contained in five Tetralysal 300 tablets. Each tablet contains 408 mg lymecycline equivalent to 300 mg tetracycline.

10   The amount of amoxicillin trihydrate required to prepare 10 capsules each containing 250 mg amoxicillin. (RMM: amoxicillin, $C_{16}H_{19}N_3O_5S$ = 365.4 g/mol; amoxicillin trihydrate, $C_{16}H_{19}N_3O_5S.3H_2O$ = 419.4 g/mol.)

Directions for Questions 11 and 12. The questions in this section are followed by three responses. ONE or MORE of the responses is (are) correct. Decide which of the responses is (are) correct. Then choose:

Directions summarised:				
A 1, 2, 3	B 1, 2 only	C 2, 3 only	D 1 only	E 3 only

11   Diclofenac tablets contain 50 mg diclofenac sodium. (RMM: diclofenac, $C_{14}H_{11}Cl_2NO_2$ = 296.1 g/mol; diclofenac sodium, $C_{14}H_{10}Cl_2NO_2.Na$ = 318.1 g/mol.)
    Which of the following is/are correct?

1 100 tablets contain 46.54 g diclofenac

2 10 g diclofenac sodium would be required to prepare 200 tablets

3 636.4 g diclofenac sodium contains 2 mol sodium ions

12 Galfer capsules contain 305 mg ferrous fumarate. (RMM: ferrous fumarate, $C_4H_2FeO_4$ = 169.9 g/mol; iron, Fe = 55.85 g/mol.) Which of the following is/are correct?

1 The iron content of 10 Galfer capsules is 1.003 g

2 76.25 g ferrous fumarate would be required to prepare 250 Galfer capsules

3 5 mol iron are contained in 8.495 kg ferrous fumarate

Directions for Questions 13–19. In this section, each question or incomplete statement is followed by five suggested answers. Select the best answer in each case.

13 Tablets containing 50 mg cortisone acetate have been formulated. Which of the following is the amount of steroid in each tablet? (RMM: cortisone, $C_{21}H_{28}O_5$ = 360.4 g/mol; cortisone acetate, $C_{23}H_{30}O_6$ = 402.5 g/mol.)

    A   36.04 g
    B   40.25 g
    C   44.77 g
    D   22.39 g
    E   45.00 g

14 Which of the following is the amount of erythromycin lactobionate in a vial containing the equivalent of 500 mg erythromycin for reconstitution? (RMM: erythromycin, $C_{37}H_{67}NO_{13}$ = 733.9 g/mol; erythromycin lactobionate, $C_{37}H_{67}NO_{13}.C_{12}H_{22}O_{12}$ = 1092.2 g/mol.)

    A   604.12 mg
    B   500.00 mg
    C   1.49 g
    D   7.44 g
    E   744.11 mg

15 An experimental antidepressant is found to undergo a first-order degradation reaction when formulated as an aqueous solution. The first-order degradation reaction has a half-life of 1.98 days. Given that the half-life, $t_{1/2}$, of a first-order reaction is described by the equation $t_{1/2} = 0.693/k$, where k is the experimentally determined first-order rate constant, which of the following is the rate constant for this reaction?

    A   1.37 days^{-1}
    B   1972.80 min^{-1}
    C   0.35 day^{-1}
    D   0.35 mol day
    E   0.35 mol

16 The enzyme-catalysed breakdown of drug A (RMM = 470 g/mol) to yield degradation product B (RMM = 235 g/mol) is known to follow zero-order kinetics. The concentration of B after 2 h of reaction is 23.5 mg/L. The amount of product, x, formed by a zero-order reaction is given by $x = kt$, where k is the experimentally determined zero-order rate constant and t is the time after the start of the reaction. Which of the following is the zero-order rate constant for this reaction?

    A   11.75 g/L per h
    B   47.00 mg/L per h
    C   0.05 mmol/h
    D   0.20 mmol/h
    E   0.20 h

17 Which of the following is the number of moles of 5-aminolevulinic acid hydrochloride in 50 mL of a 1 mol/L solution?

    A   0.005 mol
    B   0.5 mol
    C   0.25 mol
    D   0.05 mol
    E   0.025 mol

18 Which of the following is the percentage of lithium in 200 mg lithium carbonate? (RMM: lithium carbonate, Li_2CO_3 = 73.89 g/mol; lithium, Li = 6.941 g/mol.)

    A   18.79%
    B   9.39%
    C   0.94%

D 1.88%
E 2.05%

19 Which of the following is the number of millimoles of water in 1000 mg calcium chloride hexahydrate? (RMM: calcium chloride hexahydrate, $CaCl_2.6H_2O$ = 219 g/mol; water: H_2O = 18 g/mol.)

A 18.6 mmol
B 54.8 mmol
C 13.7 mmol
D 82.6 mmol
E 27.4 mmol

Directions for Questions 20–22 For each numbered question, select the one lettered option that is most closely related to it. Within the group of questions, each lettered option may be used once, more than once or not at all.
Questions 20–22 concern the following quantities:

A 3.74 mol
B 5.00 mmol
C 2.50 mmol
D 2.87 mol
E 5.03 mmol

Select, from A to E above, which is appropriate:

20 The amount of pyrazine, 2,5-dipropionic acid (PY), produced when 5 mmol 5-aminolevulinic acid (ALA) completely degrades at pH 10 according to the following reaction:
2ALA → PY

21 The number of moles in 200 g ammonium chloride. (RMM of ammonium chloride, NH_4Cl = 53.492 g/mol.)

22 The number of millimoles of potassium ions contained in 5 mL of a syrup containing 7.5% w/v potassium chloride. (RMM of: potassium chloride = 74.55 g/mol; potassium = 39.1 g/mol.)

Directions for Questions 23 and 24. The questions in this section are followed by three responses. **ONE** or **MORE** of the responses is (are) correct. Decide which of the responses is (are) correct. Then choose:

Directions summarised:

A	B	C	D	E
1, 2, 3	1, 2 only	2, 3 only	1 only	3 only

23 Betamethasone is typically included in formulated products as one of its chemical derivatives. (RMM of: betamethasone acetate, $C_{24}H_{31}FO_6$ = 434.488 g/mol; betamethasone dipropionate, $C_{28}H_{37}FO_7$ = 504.576 g/mol; betamethasone valerate, $C_{27}H_{37}FO_6$ = 476.566 g/mol.)
Which of the following is/are correct?

  1   40 g betamethasone acetate contain an equivalent amount of betamethasone as 46.4 g betamethasone dipropionate
  2   476.566 g betamethasone valerate contains 1 mol betamethasone
  3   2.5 mol betamethasone acetate weighs 1.08622 kg

24 Aminophylline is a complex of theophylline and ethylenediamine. It is typically included in pharmaceutical products as the dihydrate. (RMM of: theophylline, $C_7H_8N_4O_2$ = 180.2 g/mol; aminophylline, $(C_7H_8N_4O_2)_2.C_2H_8N_2$ = 420.5 g/mol; aminophylline dihydrate: $(C_7H_8N_4O_2)_2.C_2H_8N_2.2H_2O$ = 456.5 g/mol.)
Which of the following is/are correct?

  1   A tablet containing 100 mg aminophylline contains 108.6 mg aminophylline dihydrate
  2   A tablet containing 100 mg aminophylline contains 42.86 mg theophylline
  3   A tablet containing 100 mg aminophylline contains 10.9 mg water

Directions for Questions 25–31. In this section, each question or incomplete statement is followed by five suggested answers. Select the best answer in each case.

Questions 25 and 26. The relationship between the absorbance of ultraviolet light by a drug molecule in solution and its concentration in that solution is given by $A = \varepsilon bc$, where A is the absorbance, ε is the molar absorptivity of the drug, b the pathlength of the cell used for measurement in a spectrometer and c the concentration of the drug in solution.

25 An experimental anxiolytic agent has a molar absorptivity of 0.56 mol L/cm at 265 nm when in aqueous solution. If the pathlength of the cell used for measurement is 1 cm and the measured absorbance is 0.14, which of the following is the concentration of the drug in solution?

- A   5.00 mol/L
- B   0.05 mol/L
- C   0.25 mol/L
- D   2.50 mol/L
- E   0.50 mol/L

26 An 0.02 mol/L aqueous solution of a novel photosensitising compound has an absorbance of 0.5. Which of the following is the molar absorptivity of this compound if the pathlength of the cell used for measurement is 1 cm?

- A   25 mol L/cm⁻
- B   500 mol L/cm
- C   5 mol L/cm
- D   250 mol L/cm
- E   50 mol L/cm

Questions 27 and 28. Internal standards are often used in high-performance liquid chromatography (HPLC) to allow more robust determination of unknown drug concentrations. The ratio of peak areas (area of the sample peak/area of the internal standard peak), known as the peak area ratio, allows the unknown drug concentration to be calculated by cross-multiplication, knowing the concentration of the internal standard. A known volume of an internal standard solution of known concentration is typically added to a known volume of sample of unknown concentration and then injected onto the HPLC system for separation and analysis.

27 The peak area ratio for a HPLC analysis of hexylaminolevulinate using 5-aminolevulinic acid as internal standard is found to be 0.5. If the concentration of 5-aminolevulinic acid in the internal standard solution is 20 micrograms/mL, and 2.5 mL of this solution is added to 2.5 mL of the sample solution, which of the following is the concentration of hexylaminolevulinate in the sample solution?

    A   10.0 micrograms/mL
    B   5.0 micrograms/mL
    C   0.1 microgram/mL
    D   0.5 microgram/mL
    E   100.0 micrograms/mL

28 The peak area ratio for a HPLC analysis of uracil using phenol as an internal standard is found to be 2.5. If the concentration of phenol in the internal standard solution is 100 micrograms/mL, and 1 mL of this solution is added to 1 mL of the sample solution, which of the following is the concentration of uracil in the sample solution?

    A   25.0 micrograms/mL
    B   500.0 micrograms/mL
    C   250.0 micrograms/mL
    D   0.5 microgram/mL
    E   50.0 micrograms/mL

29 The theoretical yield for a particular route to hexylaminolevulinate synthesis is 25 g. If 18.5 g are produced, which of the following is the percentage yield for this synthetic route?

    A   74.0%
    B   7.4%
    C   18.5%
    D   25.0%
    E   60.5%

30 If the percentage yield of salbutamol sulphate produced by an industrial process is known to be 85% and 40 kg of the drug should be produced in theory, which of the following is the amount of the drug actually produced by this process?

    A   38 kg
    B   18 kg
    C   30 kg
    D   34 kg
    E   28 kg

31 The half-life for the first-order decomposition of an experimental antibiotic in aqueous solution is found to be 14 days at 20°C. If the original concentration of the drug in solution was 125 mg/5 mL, which of the following is the concentration remaining after 42 days' storage at 20°C.

    A   30.450 mg/5 mL
    B   18.450 mg/5 mL
    C   31.250 mg/5 mL
    D   62.500 mg/5 mL
    E   15.625 mg/5 mL

Directions for Questions 32–34 For each numbered question, select the one lettered option that is most closely related to it. Within the group of questions, each lettered option may be used once, more than once or not at all.
Questions 32–34 concern the following:

    A   6.25 mmol/L
    B   5.00 mmol/L
    C   12.00 mmol/L per h
    D   24.56 mmol/L per h
    E   72.00 mmol/L

Select, from A to E above, which is appropriate:

32 The zero-order rate constant for the nickel-catalysed breakdown of drug A to yield drug C if the breakdown reaction is known to follow zero-order kinetics and the concentration of C after 1 hour of reaction is 12 mmol/L. The zero-order rate equation is given by $x = kt$, where x is the concentration of product at time t and k is the experimentally determined zero-order rate constant.

33 The concentration of the single degradation product of an experimental antipsychotic 3 h after the start of the degradation reaction if the drug degrades by zero-order kinetics with an experimentally determined zero-order rate constant of 24 mmol/L per h.

34 The concentration of drug D remaining after 200 days' storage at 5°C if the half-life for the first-order decomposition of drug D in an aqueous injection formulation is found to be 50 days at 5°C and the original concentration of the drug in solution was 100 mmol/L.

Directions for Questions 35 and 36. The questions in this section are followed by three responses. **ONE** or **MORE** of the responses is (are) correct. Decide which of the responses is (are) correct. Then choose:

Directions summarised:				
A	B	C	D	E
1, 2, 3	1, 2 only	2, 3 only	1 only	3 only

35 A solution of an experimental antihypertensive contained 500 mg/mL when prepared. The drug was found to degrade via a first-order process, with an experimentally determined rate constant of 0.013 day^{-1}.
The half-life, $t_{1/2}$, of a first-order reaction is described by the equation $t_{1/2} = 0.693/k$, where k is the experimentally determined first-order rate constant. The shelf-life, t_{90}, of a product containing a drug that degrades by a first-order reaction is the time required for loss of 10% of the active substance and is described by the equation $t_{90} = 0.105/k$, where k is again the experimentally determined first-order rate constant.
Which of the following is/are correct?

1 The half-life of the product is 53.31 days
2 The shelf-life of the product is 8.08 days
3 After 100 days, the concentration of the drug remaining is 125 mg/mL

36 A pharmacopoeia monograph states that sulfathiazole sodium sesquihydrate should not contain more than 0.5% sulphonamide-related substances and loses not less than 6.0% and not more than 10.0% of its weight when dried to constant weight at 105°C. Which of the following is/are correct?

1 A 50 kg sample of sulfathiazole sodium sesquihydrate found to contain 250 mg of sulphonamide-related substances satisfies the requirements of the monograph
2 A sample of sulfathiazole sodium sesquihydrate originally weighing 2 kg is dried at 105°C to a constant weight of 1.94 kg. This does not satisfy the requirements of the monograph
3 A sample of sulfathiazole sodium sesquihydrate originally weighing 5 kg is dried at 105°C to a constant weight of 4 kg. This satisfies the requirements of the monograph

Directions for Questions 37–43. In this section, each question or incomplete statement is followed by five suggested answers. Select the best answer in each case.

Questions 37 and 38. In ultraviolet spectroscopic determination of drug concentration external standards are often employed. The absorbance at a given wavelength of a solution of known concentration is measured and then the absorbance of a sample solution of unknown concentration is then measured at the same wavelength. As absorbance at a given wavelength increases linearly with concentration, cross-multiplication allows the unknown concentration to be calculated.

37 Which of the following is the concentration of an alcoholic solution of an experimental steroid if its absorbance at 285 nm is 0.1, given that an alcoholic solution of 0.25 mg/mL has an absorbance of 0.5 at 285 nm?

    A   0.5 mg/mL
    B   0.01 mg/mL
    C   0.05 mg/mL
    D   0.10 mg/mL
    E   0.15 mg/mL

38 Which of the following is the concentration of an aqueous solution of an experimental bronchodilator if its absorbance at 230 nm is 0.25, given that an aqueous solution of 0.4 mg/mL has an absorbance of 0.1 at 230 nm?

    A   0.05 mg/mL
    B   0.01 mg/mL
    C   0.10 mg/mL
    D   0.15 mg/mL
    E   1.5 mg/mL

39 A batch of fluoxetine hydrochloride is found to contain 98% w/w of the active substance and 2% w/w impurities. Which of the following is the amount of fluoxetine hydrochloride if the batch size is 20 kg?

    A   0.4 kg
    B   19.6 kg
    C   9.8 kg

D   0.8 kg
E   15.6 kg

40 A 40 kg batch of triamterene is found to contain 39 kg of the active
    drug. What is the percentage purity of this batch?

    A   90.5%
    B   88.5%
    C   95.0%
    D   99.5%
    E   97.5%

41 An ^{131}I-labelled rose Bengal sodium injection has a radioactivity of 275
    microcuries (μCi). Given that 1 millicurie (mCi) is equal to 37
    megabecquerels (MBq), which of the following is the activity of the
    injection in megabecquerels?

    A   10.175 MBq
    B   20.350 MBq
    C   0.235 MBq
    D   0.180 MBq
    E   1.175 MBq

Questions 42 and 43 The half-life of a radioisotope can be calculated
as: $t_{1/2} = 0.693/\lambda$, where λ is the disintegration constant.

42 The disintegration constant for a radioisotope is 0.040 days^{-1}. Which
    of the following is the half-life of this radioisotope?

    A   17.325 days
    B   17.325 min
    C   34.650 min
    D   3.465 days
    E   1.175 days

43 The half-life of ^{125}I is 60 days. Which of the following is its
    disintegration constant?

    A   17.325 days
    B   18.825 min^{-1}
    C   0.012 day^{-1}
    D   3.465 days
    E   1.805 days^{-1}

Directions for Questions 44–46 For each numbered question, select the one lettered option that is most closely related to it. Within the group of questions, each lettered option may be used once, more than once or not at all.

A sample of ^{131}I has an initial activity of 60 microcuries. Its half-life is 8.08 days. The half-life of a radioisotope can be calculated as: $t_{1/2} = 0.693/\lambda$, where λ is the disintegration constant. It is known that 1 mCi = 37 MBq.

Questions 44–46 concern the following:

- A   2.22 MBq
- B   5.805 days^{-1}
- C   0.086 days^{-1}
- D   12.000 microcuries
- E   0.555 MBq

Select, from A to E above, which is appropriate:

44 The disintegration constant for this sample of ^{131}I.

45 The initial activity of this sample of ^{131}I in megabequerels.

46 The activity of the sample after storage for 24.24 days.

Directions for Questions 47 and 48. The questions in this section are followed by three responses. **ONE** or **MORE** of the responses is (are) correct. Decide which of the responses is (are) correct. Then choose:

Directions summarised:

A	B	C	D	E
1, 2, 3	1, 2 only	2, 3 only	1 only	3 only

47 Which of the following is/are correct?

1   A 50 kg batch of imiquimod with a purity of 98% contains 1.5 kg impurities

2   A reaction produces 10.5 g methylaminolevulinate. If the theoretical yield is 12 g, then the percentage yield is 88.25%

3   A 20 kg batch bendroflumethiazide is found to contain 19 kg
of the active drug. The percentage purity of this batch is 95%

48 Theophylline is released from a hydrogel-based delivery system in a
zero-order fashion, such that the amount of drug, x, released after time,
t, is given by $x = kt$, where k is the zero-order rate constant for this
release process. Which of the following is/are correct?

1   If the zero-order rate constant is 4 mmol/L per h, then 24
mmol/L of theophylline are released after 6 h
2   If 80 mmol/L are released after 24 h, then the zero-order rate
constant is 1920 mmol/L per h
3   If the zero-order rate constant is 20 mmol/L per h, then 40
mmol/L of theophylline are released after 4 h

Directions for Questions 49–55. In this section, each question or
incomplete statement is followed by five suggested answers. Select the best
answer in each case.

Questions 49 and 50. Drug A breaks down spontaneously to give
degradation product B according o the balanced stoichiometric equation
below:
A → 2B

49 Which of the following is the amount of B formed when 15 mmol A
spontaneously breaks down?

A   3.0 mmol
B   10.5 mmol
C   30.0 mmol
D   7.5 mmol
E   15.0 mmol

50 If 10 mmol B are formed, which of the following is the amount of A
that has spontaneously broken down?

A   50 mmol
B   0.1 mmol
C   5.0 mmol
D   10.0 mmol
E   0.5 mmol

Questions 51–54 It is known that, in order to convert from degrees Celsius (°C) to degrees Fahrenheit (°F) the following equation must be employed: [°C] = ([°F] − 32) × 5/9.

51 A reaction involved in the synthesis of an experimental anthelmintic requires heating to 350°F. However, the thermometer in the laboratory is marked out in degrees Celsius. Which of the following is the correct temperature for the reaction in degrees Celsius?

    A   17.67°C
    B   176.67°C
    C   572.40°C
    D   190.02°C
    E   57.24°C

52 For drug stability purposes, Daktacort cream requires storage at 2–8°C in a dispensary refrigerator. Which of the following is this temperature range expressed in degrees Fahrenheit?

    A   35.6–46.4°F
    B   82.4–95.6°F
    C   3.6–4.6°F
    D   8.2–9.6°F
    E   20.0–80.0°F

53 A candidate antiretroviral drug is found to decompose spontaneously at 120°F. Which of the following expresses in degrees centigrade this decomposition temperature?

    A   48.89°C
    B   80.12°C
    C   158.40°C
    D   8.01°C
    E   4.89°C

54 Which of the following is the boiling pint of water (100°C) expressed in degree Fahrenheit?

    A   100.00°F
    B   87.56°F
    C   300.00°F
    D   180.00°F
    E   212.00°F

55 Codeine phosphate oral solution contains 0.5% w/v codeine phosphate hemihydrate or an equivalent concentration of codeine phosphate sesquihydrate. (RMM: codeine phosphate hemihydrate, $C_{18}H_{21}NO_3.H_3PO_4.^1/_2H_2O$ = 406.4 g/mol; codeine phosphate sesquihydrate, $C_{18}H_{21}NO_3.H_3PO_4.1^1/_2H_2O$ = 424.4 g/mol.) Which of the following is the amount of codeine phosphate sesquihydrate required to prepare 500 mL codeine phosphate oral solution?

A 0.52 g
B 5.22 g
C 2.50 g
D 2.61 g
E 2.95 g

Directions for Questions 56–58 For each numbered question, select the one lettered option that is most closely related to it. Within the group of questions, each lettered option may be used once, more than once or not at all.

The half-life, $t_{1/2}$, of a first-order reaction is described by the equation $t_{1/2}$ = 0.693/k, where k is the experimentally determined first-order rate constant. The shelf life, t_{90}, of a product containing a drug that degrades by a first-order reaction is the time required for loss of 10% of the active substance and is described by the equation t_{90} = 0.105/k, where k is again the experimentally determined first-order rate constant.

Questions 56–58 concern the following:

A 0.22 years
B 5.805 h^{-1}
C 2.92 years
D 43.31 years
E 0.014 h^{-1}

Select, from A to E above, which is appropriate:

56 The experimentally determined rate constant for a first-order drug degradation reaction with a half-life of 48 h.

57 The half-life of a first-order reaction with an experimentally determined rate constant of 0.016 year^{-1}.

58 The shelf-life of a candidate oral solution containing a drug that degrades via a first-order reaction with an experimentally determined rate constant of 0.036 year^{-1}.

Directions for Questions 59 and 60. The questions in this section are followed by three responses. **ONE** or **MORE** of the responses is (are) correct. Decide which of the responses is (are) correct. Then choose:

Directions summarised:				
A 1, 2, 3	B 1, 2 only	C 2, 3 only	D 1 only	E 3 only

59 Which of the following is/are correct?

1 A 1 in 125 solution of toluidine blue O is required to carry out a chemical reaction. If 40.0 mg of the drug is dissolved and made up to a final volume of 5.0 mL, the correct concentration will have been achieved

2 6.4 g of an esterase enzyme is required to make 800.0 mL of a 0.8% w/v solution for use as a catalyst in a reaction mixture

3 A 1 in 250 solution of hexylaminolevulinate is produced by chemical synthesis. This equates to a concentration of 1.6% w/v

60 The formula for a reaction mixture is:
5-Aminolevulinic acid hydrochloride 60 mg
Methanol 3 mL
Water to 5.0 mL
Which of the following is/are correct?

1 The concentration of 5-aminolevulinic acid hydrochloride in the reaction mixture before the start of the reaction is 20 mg/mL

2 250 mL of the reaction mixture contains 150 mL methanol before the start of the reaction

3 15 mL of the reaction mixture contains 180 mg 5-aminolevulinic acid hydrochloride before the start of the reaction

ANSWERS

1 D
Ferrous gluconate tablets contain 35 mg iron/tablet, so the total daily dose is 70 mg
Plesmet syrup contains 25 mg iron/5 mL = 5 mg/mL
70/5 = 14 mL or 7 mL twice daily.
Accordingly, the correct answer is D.

2 D
The fraction of active substance per tablet is 6/7
If we divide 420 kg by 7, we get 60 kg
Multiplying by 6 gives 360 kg, the amount of active substance required.
The correct answer is therefore D.

3 A
If there are 50 mmol/L, then there are 5 mmol in 100 mL and 15 mmol in 300 mL
1 mol sodium chloride weighs 58.5 g
so 1 mmol weighs 58.5/1000 = 0.0585 g
15 mmol weighs $0.0585 \times 15 = 0.8775$ g, which can be rounded to 0.878 g.
The correct answer is A.

4 C
Calculate 10% of 350 mg, as 35 mg
Then subtract this from 350 mg to get the lower limit, 315 mg, and add it to 350 mg to get 385 mg, the upper limit.
The correct answer is C.

5 B
314.4:150
350.9:x
Cross-multiplying, $x = 167.41$
167.41 mg ranitidine hydrochloride is needed in each tablet.
The correct answer is B.

6 C
There are 150 mmol each of Na^+ and Cl^-/L of 0.9% w/v NaCl IV infusion
So, in 100 mL, you have 15 mmol

Therefore, in 50 mL you have 7.5 mmol.
The correct answer is, therefore, C.

7 B
Ferrous gluconate tablets each contain 35 mg iron, so two tablets contain 70 mg
Galfer syrup contains 45 mg iron/5 mL = 9 mg/mL
70/9 = 7.77 mL, which can be rounded to 7.8 mL.
Accordingly, the correct answer is B.

8 C
RMM of sodium chloride is 58.5
Number of moles NaCl in 500 mL of a 0.1 mol/L solution = 0.05
Accordingly, the amount of sodium chloride required = (0.05×58.5) = 2.925 g.
The correct answer is C.

9 A
This is a case of simple multiplication. 408 mg $\times$ 5 = 2040 mg, or 2.04 g.
The correct answer is A.

10 D
In 10 capsules, there will be 250 mg $\times$ 10 = 2500 mg, or 2.5 g amoxicillin
amoxicillin:amoxicillin trihydrate
365.4:419.4
2.5:x
Cross-multiplying, we have 1048.5 = $(365.4)x$
x = 2.87 g.
The correct answer is D.

11 C
1   Diclofenac:diclofenac sodium
    296.1:318.1
    x:50
    Cross-multiplying, we have: 14 805 = $(318.1)\, x$
    x = 46.54 mg
    This is the amount of diclofenac in one tablet
    Accordingly, the amount of diclofenac in 100 tablets is 4654 mg or 4.654 g.

2   There is 50 mg diclofenac sodium in one tablet, so 200 tablets must contain 200 × 50 mg = 10 000 mg, or 10 g.
3   636.4 g diclofenac sodium is equivalent to 2 mol diclofenac sodium. As diclofenac and sodium are in a molar ratio of 1:1 in diclofenac sodium, 636.4 g diclofenac sodium contains 2 mol sodium ions.
Accordingly, 2 and 3 only are true and so the correct answer is C.

12 B
1   Ferrous fumarate:iron
    169.9:55.85
    3050:x
    Cross-multiplying, we have: 170 342.5 = (169.9)x
    x = 1002.6 mg iron, or 1.003 g.
2   This is a case of simple multiplication:
    305 mg × 250 = 76 250 mg, or 76.25 g.
3   Each mole of ferrous fumarate contains 1 mol iron
    The number of moles of ferrous fumarate in 8.495 kg, or 8495 g
    8495/169.9 = 50.
Accordingly, only 1 and 2 are true and so the correct answer is B.

13 C
Cortisone:cortisone acetate
360.4:402.5
x:50
Cross-multiplying, we have (402.5)x = 18 020
x = 44.77 g.
Accordingly, the correct answer is C.

14 E
Erythromycin:erythromycin lactobionate
733.9:1092.2
500:x
Cross-multiplying, we have 546 100 = (733.9)x
x = 744.11 mg, which is the amount of erythromycin lactobionate in the vial.
The correct answer is E.

15 C
$t_{1/2} = 0.693/k$

$1.98 = 0.693/k$
$k = 0.35 \text{ day}^{-1}$
k can also be expressed as 504 min^{-1}
This is obtained by multiplying the answer above by 24 h, then 60 min.
The correct answer is C.

16 C
$x = kt$
$23.5 \text{ mg/L} = k(2 \text{ h})$
$k = 11.75 \text{ mg/L per h}$
As we have the RMM of degradation product B, we can convert the units
to millimoles per hour
$11.75 \text{ mg/L per h}/235\,000 \text{ mg/mol} = 5 \times 10^{-5} \text{ mol/h}$, or 0.05 mmol/h
The correct answer is, therefore, C.

17 D
A 1 mol/L (molar) solution contains 1 mol in 1 L
In 500 mL there are 0.5 mol and, in 50 mL, 0.05 mol.
The correct answer is D.

18 B
Lithium carbonate:lithium
73.89:6.941
200:x
Cross-multiplying, we have $1388.2 = (73.89)x$
$x = 18.79$ mg lithium in 200 mg lithium carbonate
$18.79/200 \times 100 = 9.39\%$.
The correct answer is B.

19 E
$1000 \text{ mg} = 1.0 \text{ g}$
$1.0/219 = 4.57 \times 10^{-3}$ mol calcium chloride hexahydrate
As each mole of calcium chloride hexahydrate contains 6 mol water, we
multiply by 6 to calculate the number of moles of water as: $6 \times 4.57 \times 10^{-3}$
$= 0.0274 \text{ mol}$, or 27.40 mmol.
The correct answer is E.

20 C
From the balanced stoichiometric equation, 2 mol ALA react to yield 1 mol

PY; 5 mol will, therefore, react to yield 2.5 mol PY. Dividing by 1000 gives the correct answer as 2.5 mmol.
This corresponds to option C.

21 A
200/53.492 = 3.74 mol.
The correct answer is A.

22 E
A 7.5% w/v solution contains 7.5 g in 100 mL, or 0.375 g in 5 mL
$0.375/74.5 = 5.03 \times 10^{-3}$ mol KCl in 5 mL
This equates to 5.03 mmol
1 mol KCL contains 1 mol potassium ions.
So the correct answer is E.

23 A
1   Work out the number of moles of each derivative
    Betamethasone acetate: 40/434.488 = 0.092
    Betamethasone dipropionate: 46.4/504.576 = 0.092
    Both amounts contain the same number of moles, so there is equivalence in terms of betamethasone content.
2   476.566 is the RMM of betamethasone valerate. This amount of drug is equivalent to 1 mol.
3   $434.488 \times 2.5 = 1086.22$ g or 1.08622 kg
Accordingly, all three statements are true and so the correct answer is A

24 D
1   Aminophylline:aminophylline dihydrate
    420.5:456.5
    100:x
    Cross-multiplying, we have 45 650 = (420.5)x
    $x = 108.56$
    This can be rounded to 108.6 mg aminophylline dihydrate
2   Aminophylline:theophylline
    420.5:2(180.2) = 420.5:360.4
    100:x
    Cross-multiplying, we have 36 040 = (420.5)x
    $x = 85.7$ mg theophylline.
3   Aminophylline:water
    420.5:2(18.016) = 420.5:36.032

100:x

Cross-multiplying, we have 3603.2 = (420.5)x

x = 8.57 mg water.

Accordingly, 1 only is true, so the correct answer is D.

25 C

$A = \varepsilon bc$

0.14 = 0.56 × 1 × c

0.14 = (0.56)c

c = 0.25 mol/L.

The correct answer is C.

26 D

$A = \varepsilon bc$

0.5 = ε × 1 × 0.02

0.5 = (0.02)ε

ε = 250 mol L/cm.

The correct answer is D.

27 A

Peak area ratio = concentration ratio

We need to divide the concentration by 2, because it has undergone a 1 in 2 dilution

0.5 = x/10

Multiplying both sides by 10

x = 5 micrograms/mL

We now need to multiply this concentration by 2 to take account of the 1 in 2 dilution

We now have the hexylaminolevulinate concentration in the sample as 10 micrograms/mL.

The correct answer is A.

28 C

Peak area ratio = concentration ratio

We need to divide the concentration of uracil by 2, because it has undergone a 1 in 2 dilution

2.5 = x/50

Multiplying both sides by 50

x = 125 micrograms/mL

We now need to multiply this concentration by 2 to take account of the 1 in 2 dilution
We now have the uracil concentration in the sample as 250 micrograms/mL.
The correct answer is C.

29 B
This is a case of simple multiplication and division:
18.5/25 = 0.74
0.74 × 100 = 74% yield.
Accordingly, the correct answer is B.

30 D
This is a case of simple multiplication and division.
100%:40 kg
85%:x kg
Cross-multiplying, we have: 3400 = (100) x
x = 34 kg.
The correct answer is D.

31 E
With each half-life, half of the drug is destroyed, so in 42 days, we go through three half-lives
125 mg/5 mL → 62.5 mg/5 mL → 31.25 mg/5 mL → 15.625 mg/5 mL.
Accordingly, the correct answer is E.

32 C
$x = kt$ for zero–order rate equation
12 = k(1)
k = 12 mmol/L per h.
The correct answer is C.

33 E
$x = kt$ for zero-order rate equation
x = (24)(3)
x = 72 mmol/L.
The correct answer is E.

34 A
With each half-life, half of the drug is destroyed
In 200 days, we go through four half-lives:

100 mmol/L → 50 mmol/L → 25 mmol/L → 12.5 mmol/L → 6.25 mmol/L.
Accordingly, the correct answer is A.

35 B

1     $t_{1/2} = 0.693/k$
      $= 0.693/0.013$
      $= 53.31$ days.
2     $t_{90} = 0.105/k$
      $= 0.105/0.013$
      $= 8.08$ days.
3   The concentration 125 mg/mL will be reached after two half-lives, which is 106.62 days.

Accordingly, only 1 and 2 are true, so the correct answer is B.

36 D

1   50 kg = 50 000 g
      250 mg = 0.25 g
      $(0.25/50\,000) \times 100 = 0.0005\%$
      The level of related substances is below the specified limit of 0.5%, so this sample satisfies the requirements of the monograph.
2   2 − 1.94 = 0.06 kg
      $(0.06/2) \times 100 = 3\%$ loss on drying. This sample satisfies the requirements of the monograph.
3   5 − 4 = 1 kg
      $(1/5) \times 100 = 20\%$ loss on drying. This sample does not satisfy the requirements of the monograph.

Accordingly, only 1 is true and so the correct answer is D.

37 C

0.5:0.25
0.1:x
Cross-multiplying, we have: $0.025 = (0.5)x$
$x = 0.05$ mg/mL.
The correct answer is C.

38 C

0.1:0.4
0.25:x
Cross-multiplying, we have: $0.1 = (0.1)x$

x = 1.0 mg/mL.
The correct answer is C.

39 B
(20/100) × 98 = 19.6 kg fluoxetine hydrochloride.
The correct answer is B.

40 E
(39/40) × 100 = 97.5% purity.
The correct answer is E.

41 A
275 microcuries = 0.275 mCi
1 mCi = 37 MBq
0.275 mCi = x MBq
Cross-multiplying, we have: 10.175 = x
x = 10.175 MBq.
The correct answer is A.

42 A
$t_{1/2}$ = 0.693/λ
= 0.693/0.040
= 17.325 days.
The correct answer is A.

43 C
$t_{1/2}$ = 0.693/λ
60 = 0.693/λ
(60)λ = 0.693
= 0.01155 day^{-1}
This can be rounded to 0.012 day^{-1}.
The correct answer is C.

44 C
$t_{1/2}$ = 0.693/λ
8.08 = 0.693/λ
(8.08)λ = 0.693
= 0.0858 day^{-1}
This can be rounded to 0.086 day^{-1}.
The correct answer is C.

45 A
60 microcuries = 0.06 mCi
1 mCi = 37 MBq
0.06 mCi = x MBq
Cross-multiplying, we have: 2.22 = x
x =2.22 MBq.
The correct answer is A.

46 E
$8.08 \times 3 = 24.24$ = three half-lives
The activity will go from 60 microcuries to 30 microcuries to 15 microcuries in this time
There is no answer corresponding to 15 microcuries; converting to megabecquerels:
15 microcuries = 0.015 mCi
1 mCi = 37 MBq
0.015 mCi = x MBq
Cross-multiplying, we have: 0.555 = x
x = 0.555 MBq.
The correct answer is E.

47 E
1    $(50/100) \times 2 = 1$ kg impurities
2    $(10.5/12) \times 100 = 87.5\%$ = the percentage yield
3    $(19/20) \times 100 = 95\%$ = the percentage purity of the batch.
Accordingly, only 3 is true and so the correct answer is E.

48 D
1    $x = kt$
     $= 4(6)$
     $= 24$ mmol/L.
2    $x = kt$
     $80 = k(24)$
     $k = 3.33$ mmol/L per h.
3    $x = kt$
     $= 20(4)$
     $= 80$ mmol/L.
Accordingly, only 1 is true and so the correct answer is D.

49 C
From the balanced stoichiometric equation above, 1 mol A reacts to yield 2 mol B
15 mol will, therefore, react to yield 30 mol B
Dividing by 1000 gives the correct answer as 30 mmol.
The correct answer is C.

50 C
From the balanced stoichiometric equation above, 1 mol A reacts to yield 2 mol B
If 10 mol B were formed, then 5 mol A would have spontaneously broken down
Dividing by 1000 gives the correct answer as 5 mmol.
The correct answer is C.

51 B
$[°C] = ([°F] - 32) \times 5/9$
$= (350 - 32) \times 5/9$
$= (318) \times 5/9$
$= 176.67°C.$
The correct answer is B.

52 A
$[°C] = ([°F] - 32) \times 5/9$
$2 = (x - 32) \times 5/9$
Dividing across by 5/9, we have:
$3.6 = x - 32$
$x = 35.6°F$
$8 = (x - 32) \times 5/9$
Dividing across by 5/9, we have:
$14.4 = x - 32$
$x = 46.4°F.$
Accordingly, the correct answer is A.

53 A
$[°C] = ([°F] - 32) \times 5/9$
$= (120 - 32) \times 5/9$
$= (88) \times 5/9$
$= 48.89°C.$
The correct answer is A.

54 E
$[°C] = ([°F] - 32) \times 5/9$
$100 = (x - 32) \times 5/9$
Dividing across by 5/9, we have:
$180 = x - 32$
$x = 212°F.$
The correct answer is E.

55 D
500 mL of a 0.5% w/v solution contains 2.5 g codeine phosphate hemihydrate
We need to calculate the equivalent amount of codeine phosphate sesquihydrate
406.4:424.4
2.5:x
Cross-multiplying, we have:
$1061 = (406.4)x$
$x = 2.61$ g.
Accordingly, the correct answer is D.

56 E
$t_{1_{/2}} = 0.693/k$
$48 = 0.693/k$
$48k = 0.693$
$k = 0.014$ h^{-1}.
The correct answer is E.

57 D
$t_{1_{/2}} = 0.693/k$
$= 0.693/0.016$
$= 43.31$ years.
The correct answer is D.

58 C
$t_{90} = 0.105/k$
$= 0.105/0.036$
$= 2.92$ years.
The correct answer is C.

59 B

1   A 1 in 125 solution contains 1.0 g, or 1000.0 mg, in 125.0 mL Dividing by 25 gives 40.0 mg in 5.0 mL.

2   0.8% w/v is equivalent to 0.8 g in 100.0 mL or 6.4 g in 800.0 mL.

3   A 1 in 250 solution contains 1.0 g in 250.0 mL
(1/250) × 100 = 0.4% w/v.

Only 1 and 2 are correct, so the correct answer is B.

60 C

1   There are 60 mg 5-aminolevulinic acid hydrochloride in 5.0 mL of the reaction mixture before the start of the reaction, so there must be 12 mg in 1 mL. The concentration is 12 mg/mL.

2   5 mL of the reaction mixture contains 3 mL methanol, so multiplying both by 50 gives 150 mL methanol in 250 mL of the reaction mixture before the start of the reaction.

3   5 mL of the reaction mixture contains 60 mg 5-aminolevulinic acid hydrochloride before the start of the reaction, so 15 mL must contain 180 mg.

Accordingly, 2 and 3 are true and so the correct answer is C.

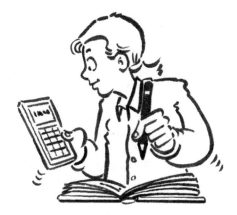

Practice tests

PRACTICE TEST 1 – QUESTIONS

> **Directions for Questions 1–14.** Each of the questions or incomplete statements in this section is followed by five suggested answers. Select the best answer in each case.

1   A child is prescribed methotrexate once weekly for leukaemia. Upon checking the patient's case notes you find that the child is 2 feet 5 inches tall and weighs 11 kg. The standard paediatric dose of methotrexate for leukaemia is 15 mg/m².

Body surface area (m²) $= \sqrt{\dfrac{\text{weight (kg)} \times \text{height (cm)}}{3600}}$

1 foot = 12 inches = 304.8 mm
Given this information, which of the following is a suitable weekly dose of methotrexate for this child?

    A   10 mg
    B   9.86 mg
    C   8.75 mg
    D   7.11 mg
    E   6.43 mg

2   Which of the following are the correct amounts of morphine sulphate contained in 150 mL Oramorph oral solution and 15 mL Oramorph concentrated oral solution?
Oramorph oral solution: morphine sulphate 10 mg/5 mL
Oramorph concentrated oral solution: morphine sulphate 100 mg/5 mL

    A   150 mg in 150 mL Oramorph oral solution and 300 mg in 15 mL Oramorph concentrated oral solution

B   15 mg in 150 mL Oramorph oral solution and 150 mg in
     15 mL Oramorph concentrated oral solution
C   15 mg in 150 mL Oramorph oral solution and 300 mg in
     15 mL Oramorph concentrated oral solution
D   150 mg in both 150 mL Oramorph oral solution and 15 mL
     Oramorph concentrated oral solution
E   300 mg in both 150 mL Oramorph oral solution and 15 mL
     Oramorph concentrated oral solution

3   An ointment contains 1% w/w calamine. How much calamine powder
    would it be appropriate to add to 200 g of the ointment to produce a
    4% w/w calamine ointment?

    A   4.25 g
    B   5.5 g
    C   6.25 g
    D   6.5 g
    E   8.25 g

4   You are asked to advise on the dose of aminophylline for a 6-year-old
    girl who weighs 44 lb. The prescriber wants to dilute 250 mg
    aminophylline in 250 mL sodium chloride 0.9% and asks you to
    calculate the infusion rate. Given that the dosage of aminophylline in
    children between the ages of 1 month and 9 years is 1 mg/kg per h,
    which of the following is the correct infusion rate? (1 kg = 2.2 lb.)

    A   10 mL/h
    B   20 mL/h
    C   25 mL/h
    D   30 mL/h
    E   40 mL/h

5   What weight of sodium bicarbonate is contained in 450 mL Aromatic
    Magnesium Carbonate Mixture, BP?
    Aromatic Magnesium Carbonate Mixture, BP: light magnesium
    carbonate 3%, sodium bicarbonate 5%, in a suitable vehicle containing
    aromatic cardamom tincture.

    A   15 g
    B   17.5 g
    C   20 g
    D   22.5 g
    E   25 g

6 A woman presents the following legally written prescription for her son who is 6 years old:
Levothyroxine 50 micrograms/5 mL oral solution – 200 micrograms daily
Dexamethasone 2 mg/5 mL oral solution – 200 micrograms every 12 h
Which of the following is the correct volume of both solutions needed to provide supplies that will last 28 days?

    A   280 mL levothyroxine 50 micrograms/5 mL oral solution and 7 mL dexamethasone 2 mg/5mL oral solution

    B   280 mL levothyroxine 50 micrograms/5 mL oral solution and 14 mL dexamethasone 2 mg/5 mL oral solution

    C   280 mL levothyroxine 50 micrograms/5 mL oral solution and 28 mL dexamethasone 2 mg/5 mL oral solution

    D   560 mL levothyroxine 50 micrograms/5 mL oral solution and 14 mL dexamethasone 2 mg/5 mL oral solution

    E   560 mL levothyroxine 50 micrograms/5 mL oral solution and 28 mL dexamethasone 2 mg/5 mL oral solution

7 A 9-year-old boy is currently using En-De-Kay daily fluoride mouth rinse under the recommendation of his dentist. The mouth rinse contains sodium fluoride at a concentration of 0.05%. What weight of sodium fluoride is contained in each 10 mL volume with which he rinses his mouth?

    A   5000 micrograms
    B   500 micrograms
    C   50 micrograms
    D   5 micrograms
    E   0.5 microgram

8 Mr P is currently taking Mucogel suspension at a daily dose of 20 mL three times daily. How much dried aluminium hydroxide will Mr P have taken after 10 days' compliant use of Mucogel?
Mucogel contains magnesium hydroxide 195 mg and dried aluminium hydroxide 220 mg/5 mL.

    A   3.9 g
    B   5.85 g
    C   7.8 g
    D   17.8 g
    E   26.4 g

9 Miss T, aged 18 years, weighs 55 kg and has a body surface area equal to 1.6 m². She has been started on CellCept suspension (mycophenolate mofetil 1 g/5 mL when reconstituted with water) following a kidney transplantation. She is taking the medicine at a dose of 600 mg/m² twice daily. How many complete days of compliant therapy will each 175 mL bottle of reconstituted CellCept suspension provide Miss T?
The shelf-life of the reconstituted suspension is 2 months.

  A   12 days
  B   17 days
  C   18 days
  D   23 days
  E   58 days

10 Mrs M is given an intravenous dose of drug K and her peak serum level is found to be 100 micrograms/mL; 2 hours later her serum concentration is found to be 1.5625 mg/L. What is the elimination half-life $(t_{1/2})$ of drug K in Mrs M? (You may assume that the distribution is complete and that the elimination is described by a first-order process.)

  A   10 min
  B   20 min
  C   30 min
  D   40 min
  E   50 min

11 Which of the following is the volume of fluoxetine (as hydrochloride) 20 mg/5 mL liquid required to be added to a suitable volume of an appropriate diluent to obtain 250 mL fluoxetine (as hydrochloride) liquid 2 mg/mL?

  A   60 mL
  B   70 mL
  C   85 mL
  D   110 mL
  E   125 mL

12 A vial containing 500 mg methylprednisolone (as sodium succinate) powder for reconstitution is reconstituted with sterile water for injection. Which of the following is the displacement value of methylprednisolone sodium succinate given that 7.8 mL sterile Water for Injection, BP is added to the powder to produce 8 mL solution?

  A   0.05 mL/g
  B   0.25 mL/g

    C   0.4 mL/g
    D   0.75 mL/g
    E   1.0 mL/g

13 The formula for morphine oral solution is:
    Morphine hydrochloride 5 mg
    Chloroform water to 5 mL
    You work in a special manufacturing unit and are requested to extemporaneously prepare 240 mL of 10 mg/5 mL morphine oral solution. Which of the following is the amount of morphine hydrochloride that you would need?

    A   0.3 g
    B   0.48 g
    C   0.6 g
    D   0.76 g
    E   0.9 g

14 A liquid medicine is supplied in a concentration of 100 mg/5 mL. A patient requires 25 mg orally four times daily for 7 days, 20 mg three times daily for 5 days, 15 mg twice daily for 3 days and then 10 mg daily thereafter. Which of the following is the volume of liquid medicine that you will need to dispense for the first 28 days of therapy?

    A   605 mL
    B   204 mL
    C   303 mL
    D   61 mL
    E   32 mL

Directions for Questions 15–18. For each numbered question select the one lettered option that is most closely related to it. Within the group of questions each lettered option may be used once, more than once, or not at all.

Question 15 concerns the following quantities:

    A   10
    B   50
    C   115
    D   165
    E   378

Select, from A to E above, which is appropriate:

15 The total number of doses available within four 125 mL bottles of mefenamic acid 50 mg/5 mL oral solution when it is prescribed at a dose of 500 mg three times daily

Questions 16–18 concern the following quantities:

    A   0.8 L
    B   1 L
    C   3 L
    D   54 L
    E   60 L

Select, from A to E above, which is appropriate:

16 The apparent volume of distribution (V_D) when a 300 mg intravenous dose of drug O produces an immediate blood concentration of 5 micrograms/mL.
Volume of distribution (V_D) can be defined as:
$V_D = D/C_p$
in which D = total amount of drug in the body, C_p = plasma concentration of drug.

17 The apparent volume of distribution (V_D) when a 0.4 kg intravenous dose of drug R produces an immediate blood concentration of 0.4 g/mL.

18 The apparent volume of distribution (V_D) when a 720 microgram intravenous dose of drug S produces an immediate blood concentration of 0.9×10^{-6} g/mL.

Directions for Questions 19 and 20. The questions in this section are followed by three responses. **ONE** or **MORE** of the responses is (are) correct. Decide which of the responses is (are) correct. Then choose:

    A   If 1, 2 and 3 are correct
    B   If 1 and 2 only are correct
    C   If 2 and 3 only are correct
    D   If 1 only is correct
    E   If 3 only is correct

Directions summarised:				
A 1, 2, 3	**B** 1, 2 only	**C** 2, 3 only	**D** 1 only	**E** 3 only

19 Which of the following is/are correct?

    1   40 mL Pholcodine Linctus, BP is required to prepare 100 mL Galenphol paediatric linctus

    2   40 mL Pholcodine Linctus, Strong, BP is required to prepare 100 mL Pholcodine Linctus, BP

    3   20 mL Pholcodine Linctus, Strong, BP is required to prepare 60 mL Galenphol paediatric linctus

Galenphol paediatric linctus: pholcodine 2 mg/5 mL oral solution
Pholcodine Linctus, BP: pholcodine 5 mg/5 mL oral solution
Pholcodine Linctus, Strong, BP: pholcodine 10 mg/5 mL oral solution

20 You are required to make an intravenous infusion with the following formulae:
Sodium bicarbonate 180 mmol/L
Potassium chloride 150 mmol/L
Sodium chloride 90 mmol/L
The molecular weights are:
Sodium bicarbonate 84
Potassium chloride 74.5
Sodium chloride 58.5
Which of the following is/are correct?

    1   15.4 g potassium chloride is required to prepare 2500 mL of this solution

    2   26.6 g sodium bicarbonate is required to prepare 4 L of this solution

    3   7.89 g is the combined weight of these three ingredients in 250 mL of this solution

PRACTICE TEST 1 – ANSWERS

1 D
First of all need to convert the height of the patient into centimetres rather than feet and inches
1 foot = 12 inches = 304.8 mm
Therefore height of child = (2 × 304.88) + (304.8/12 × 5) mm
= 609.76 mm + 127.03 mm
= 73.68 cm
Body surface area $(m^2) = \sqrt{(weight\ [kg] \times height\ [cm])/3600}$
BSA $(m^2) = \sqrt{(11 \times 73.68)/3600}$
$= \sqrt{0.225}$
$= 0.474\ m^2$
Weekly dose of methotrexate = 15 mg/m²
= 15 × 0.474 mg
= 7.11 mg.
Therefore, the correct answer is D.

2 E
Oramorph oral solution: morphine sulphate 10 mg/5 mL
10 mg morphine sulphate in 5 mL of solution
2 mg morphine sulphate in 1 mL of solution
150 × 2 mg morphine sulphate in 150 mL of solution
300 mg morphine sulphate in 150 mL of solution
Oramorph concentrated oral solution: morphine sulphate 100 mg/5 mL
100 mg of morphine sulphate in 5 mL of concentrated solution
20 mg of morphine sulphate in 1 mL of concentrated solution
15 × 20 mg of morphine sulphate in 15 mL of concentrated solution
300 mg of morphine sulphate in 15 mL of concentrated solution.
Therefore, the correct answer is E.

3 C
Original ointment strength is 1% w/w
= 1 g calamine in 100 g ointment
= 2 g of calamine in 200 g ointment
New strength = 4% w/w
= 4 g of calamine in 100 g ointment
Let *x* g = the extra amount of calamine powder added to the 200 g of 1% w/w ointment

New total weight of ointment = 200 + x g
Calamine content = 2 + x g
Strength = 4% w/w, so $(2 + x)/(200 + x) = 4/100$
$100 \times (2 + x) = 4 \times (200 + x)$
$200 + 100x = 800 + 4x$
$200 - 800 = 4x - 100x$
$-600 = -96x$
$96x = 600$
$x = 6.25$ g.
Therefore, the correct answer is C.

4 B
First of all need to convert weight of girl into kilograms:
1 kg = 2.2 lb
1 lb = 1/2.2 kg
44 lb = 44/2.2 kg = 20 kg
Dose: 1 mg/kg per h = 20 mg/h
Strength of solution being administered = 250 mg/250 mL = 1 mg/mL
Rate: 20 mg/h
1 mg in 1 mL, so 20 mg in 20 mL
20 mL/h.
Therefore, the correct answer is B.

5 D
5% of total volume is sodium bicarbonate
Total volume of 450 mL, so weight of sodium bicarbonate is 5/100 × 450
g = 22.5 g.
Therefore, the correct answer is D.

6 E
Levothyroxine 200 micrograms daily: 50 micrograms/5 mL, so 5 × 4 mL
contains 200 micrograms = 20 mL daily
Over 28 days will use 280 × 20 mL = 560 mL
Dexamethasone 200 micrograms every 12 h = 200 × 2 micrograms daily =
400 micrograms daily
2 mg/5 mL solution = 2000 micrograms/5 mL = 400 micrograms/mL, so
dose is 0.5 mL every 12 h
Over 28 days will use 0.5 × 2 × 28 mL = 28 mL.
Therefore, the correct answer is E.

7 A
0.05% = 0.05 g in 100 mL
Therefore, 0.005 g in 10 mL = 5 mg = 5000 micrograms.
Therefore, the correct answer is A.

8 E
Each dose of Mucogel suspension is 20 mL, so contains 4 × 220 mg dried aluminium hydroxide
Each day Mr P takes three doses = 4 × 220 × 3 mg dried aluminium hydroxide = 2640 mg
Therefore, she will have taken 2640 × 10 mg after 10 days
= 26 400 mg = 26.4 g.
Therefore, the correct answer is E.

9 C
Each dose = 600 mg/m^2
For Miss T = 600 × 1.6 mg = 960 mg
Therefore, each day she will use 960 × 2 mg = 1920 mg
Suspension strength is 1 g/5mL
1920 mg = 1.92 g
1.92 g in 5 × 1.92 mL = 9.6 mL
Each bottle contains 175 mL = 175/9.6 days of therapy = 18.23 days
Each bottle therefore contains enough medicine for 18 complete days of therapy.
Therefore, the correct answer is C.

10 B
Peak serum level = 100 micrograms/mL
After 2 h, serum concentration = 1.5625 mg/L
First of all need to have both concentrations in the same units:
Peak serum level = 100 000 micrograms/L
After 2 h serum concn = 1562.5 micrograms/L
The serum concentration will reduce as follows:
100 000 → 50 000 → 25 000 → 12 500 → 6250 → 3125 → 1562.5
Therefore, six half-lives have passed for serum concentration to reduce from 100 000 to 1562.5 micrograms/L
These six half-lives have taken 2 h, so each $t_{1/2}$ lasts 120/6 min = 20 min.
Therefore, the correct answer is B.

11 E
250 mL of 2 mg/mL liquid contains 2 × 250 mg fluoxetine hydrochloride
= 500 mg
Original liquid contains 20 mg/5 mL fluoxetine hydrochloride
= 4 mg/mL
Need to calculate the volume of original liquid that contains 500 mg
Volume = 500/4 = 125 mL.
Therefore, the correct answer is E.

12 C
Final volume is 8 mL and this includes 7.8 mL of sterile water for injection
and 500 mg methylprednisolone sodium succinate
Therefore 500 mg displaces 0.2 mL, so 0.2 mL/500 mg = 2 mL/5000 mg
= 0.4 mL/g.
The correct answer is C.

13 B
Strength is 10 mg/5mL, so in 240 mL the content of morphine hydrochloride
= 240/5 × 10 mg
= 480 mg
= 0.48 g.
Therefore, the correct answer is B.

14 D
Days 1–7: 25 mg four times daily = 25 × 4 × 7 mg =700 mg
Days 8–12: 20 mg three times daily = 20 × 3 × 5 mg = 300 mg
Days 13–15: 15 mg twice daily = 15 × 2 × 3 = 90 mg
Days 16–28: 10 mg daily = 10 × 13 = 130 mg
Total drug required = 1220 mg
Liquid medicine strength is 100 mg/5 mL = 1 mg/5/100 mL
1220 mg in 1220 × 5/100 mL = 61 mL.
Therefore, the correct answer is D.

15 A
Strength is 50 mg/5 mL and each dose is 500 mg, so each dose is (500/50
× 5) mL = 50 mL
Each bottle contains 125 mL, so four bottles contain 500 mL
Number of doses available is 500/50 = 10 doses.
Therefore, the correct answer is A.

16 E
D = 300 mg = 300 000 micrograms
C_p = 5 mg/mL = 5000 micrograms/L
$V_D = D/C_p$
V_D (L) = 300 000 micrograms/5000 micrograms/L
V_D = 60 L.
Therefore, the correct answer is E.

17 B
D = 0.4 kg = 400 g
C_p = 0.4 g/mL
$V_D = D/C_p$
V_D (L) = 400/0.4 = 1000 mL = 1 L.
Therefore, the correct answer is B.

18 A
D = 720 micrograms
C_p = 0.9×10^{-6} g/mL = 0.9 micrograms/mL
$V_D = D/C_p$
V_D = 720/0.9 mL = 800 mL = 0.8 L.
Therefore the correct answer is A.

19 D
1   Galenphol paediatric linctus: pholcodine 2 mg/5 mL, so 100 mL
      contains $100/5 \times 2$ mg = 40 mg
      Pholcodine Linctus, BP: pholcodine 5 mg/5 mL, so 40 mL contains
      $40/5 \times 5$ mg = 40 mg
      Therefore, this statement is true.
2   Pholcodine Linctus, Strong, BP: pholcodine 10 mg/5 mL oral solution,
      so 40 mL contains $40/5 \times 10$ mg = 80 mg
      Pholcodine Linctus, BP: pholcodine 5 mg/5 mL oral solution, so 100
      mL contains $100/5 \times 5$ mg = 100 mg
      Therefore, this statement is false.
3   Pholcodine Linctus, Strong, BP: pholcodine 10 mg/5 mL oral solution,
      so 20 mL contains $20/5 \times 10$ mg = 40 mg
      Galenphol paediatric linctus: pholcodine 2 mg/5 mL oral solution, so
      60 mL contains $60/5 \times 2$ = 24 mg
      Therefore, this statement is false.
Overall, only statement 1 is true, so the correct answer is D.

20 E

1   Potassium chloride 150 mmol/L
        1 mol potassium chloride = 74.5 g
        1 mmol potassium chloride = 74.5/1000 g = 0.0745 g
        150 mmol = 150 × 0.0745 g = 11.175 g
        Strength: potassium chloride 11.175 g/L
        2500 mL = 2.5 L
        2.5 L contains 11.175 × 2.5 = 27.9375 g
        Therefore, the statement is false.

2   Sodium bicarbonate 180 mmol/L
        1 mol sodium bicarbonate = 84 g
        1 mmol of sodium bicarbonate = 84/1000 g = 0.084 g
        180 mmol = 0.084 × 180 g = 15.12 g
        Strength: 180 mmol/L = 15.12 g/L
        4 L contains 15.12 × 4 = 60.48 g
        Therefore, the statement is false.

3   Sodium bicarbonate 180 mmol/L = 180/4 mmol in 250 mL = 45 mmol
        Potassium chloride 150 mmol/L = 150/4 mmol in 250 mL = 37.5 mmol
        Sodium chloride 90 mmol/L = 90/4 mmol in 250 mL = 22.5 mmol
        Sodium bicarbonate 45 mmol = 84 × 45/1000 g = 3.78 g
        Potassium chloride 37.5 mmol = 74.5 × 37.5/1000 g = 2.79375 g
        Sodium chloride 22.5 mmol = 58.5 × 22.5/1000 g = 1.31625 g
        Total = 3.78 + 2.79375 + 1.31625 = 7.89 g
        Therefore, the statement is true.

Overall only 3 is true, so the correct answer is E.

PRACTICE TEST 2 - QUESTIONS

Directions for Questions 1–14. Each of the questions or incomplete statements in this section is followed by five suggested answers. Select the best answer in each case.

1 A patient with diabetes uses Byetta as one of his medications. After his recent hospital review, his dose has been adjusted to 5 micrograms before lunch and 10 micrograms before his evening dinner. He currently has two unopened 5 microgram/dose prefilled pens at home and asks you how many days in total these two pens will now last him. Which of the following is the correct reply?

Byetta injection contains exenatide 250 micrograms/mL available as 5 microgram/dose and 10 microgram/dose prefilled pens, both containing 60 doses.

   A 25 days
   B 30 days
   C 35 days
   D 40 days
   E 45 days

2 You have in your pharmacy 400 mg potassium permanganate tablets. You are requested to prepare 2 L of a potassium permanganate solution such that the patient will dilute this 1 in 10 to obtain a 0.005% solution suitable for wound washing. How many of these tablets would you dissolve in a small amount of water before making the solution up to a final volume of 2 L with water?

   A 2.5 tablets
   B 3 tablets
   C 3.5 tablets
   D 4 tablets
   E 4.5 tablets

3 Mrs C has been receiving 40 mg morphine sulphate oral solution every 4 h. Her doctor now wants to change her to 24-hourly MXL (morphine sulphate modified-release) capsules. What daily dose of MXL capsules will provide an equivalent dose of morphine for Mrs C?

   A 60 mg every 24 h
   B 90 mg every 24 h

C   120 mg every 24 h
D   2 × 120 mg every 24 h
E   150 mg and 30 mg every 24 h

4   If 1200 mg potassium permanganate is dissolved in 4 L water, what is the percentage strength of the resulting solution?

A   0.003%
B   0.015%
C   0.03%
D   0.15%
E   0.3%

5   The recommended intravenous injection dose of gentamicin for the treatment of septicaemia for a child aged between 1 month and 12 years is 2.5 mg/kg every 8 h. What volume of gentamicin 40 mg/mL should be given every 8 h to a 10-year-old girl weighing 30 kg?

A   2.5 mL
B   2.225 mL
C   2.0 mL
D   1.875 mL
E   1.7 mL

6   Bernard, a 6-year-old boy (weight 20 kg) with epilepsy, currently takes Epilim liquid (sodium valproate 200 mg/5 mL) at a dose of 7.5 mg/kg twice daily. What volume of Epilim liquid will Bernard take during the month of November? You can assume that he is fully compliant and no spillages or medication loss occur during the month of November.

A   225 mL
B   350 mL
C   465 mL
D   500 mL
E   530.5 mL

7   Drug E has been prescribed for a 6-month-old baby with a body surface area of 0.42 m². Drug E should be given as a daily dose of 2 mg/m² in two divided doses. It is formulated as a syrup with a 500 microgram/mL concentration. Which of the following is an appropriate single dose of drug E syrup for this baby?

A   0.4 mL
B   0.84 mL

    C   1.68 mL
    D   8 mL
    E   40 mL

8   Drug P has an elimination rate constant (k_{el}) of 0.924 h^{-1} and displays first-order kinetics. Given that $k_{el} = 0.693/t_{1/2}$, at 12pm which of the following is the concentration of drug P in a patient, given that the peak serum concentration of drug P is 50 mg/L at 9am?

    A   0.987 micrograms/mL
    B   1.654 micrograms/mL
    C   2.31 micrograms/mL
    D   3.125 micrograms/mL
    E   4.978 micrograms/mL

9   Jelliffe's equation can be used to estimate creatinine clearance (Cl_{Cr}) in units of mL/min per 1.73 m^2. For males:

$$Cl_{Cr} = \frac{98 - 0.8 \times (\text{patient's age in years} - 20)}{\text{serum creatinine (mg/dL)}}$$

Using Jelliffe's equation what is the estimated creatinine clearance for Brian, aged 45 years, who has a serum creatinine of 3 mg/dL, weighs 65 kg and has a body surface area of 1.8 m^2

    A   Approximately 23.60 mL/min
    B   Approximately 24.89 mL/min
    C   Approximately 25.34 mL/min
    D   Approximately 26 mL/min
    E   Approximately 27.05 mL/min

10 A 1 in 5000 solution of copper sulphate contains which of the following concentrations?

    A   50 mg copper sulphate in 500 mL solution
    B   20 mg copper sulphate in 100 mL solution
    C   5 mg copper sulphate in 500 mL solution
    D   100 mg copper sulphate in 1000 mL solution
    E   50 mg copper sulphate in 300 mL solution

11 Which of the following amounts of chlorhexidine gluconate is required to make 20 mL of a stock solution, such that, when the stock solution is diluted 30 times with water, a final solution of 0.2% w/v chlorhexidine gluconate is produced?

A 0.2 g
B 0.4 g
C 0.8 g
D 1.2 g
E 1.8 g

12 A new respite patient has been admitted into one of the care homes to which you supply medication. She has been admitted into the care home for a total of 10 days. The home requires you to supply 10 days of her liquid medicines to cover her stay. She usually takes dipyridamole 300 mg daily in three divided doses and propranolol 320 mg daily. Which of the following are the correct amounts of both liquid medicines to supply for 10 days of therapy?

    A   50 mL propranolol 50 mg/5 mL oral solution and 50 mL dipyridamole 50 mg/5 mL solution

    B   100 mL propranolol 50 mg/5 mL oral solution and 50 mL dipyridamole 50 mg/5 mL solution

    C   100 mL propranolol 50 mg/5 mL oral solution and 150 mL dipyridamole 50 mg/5 mL solution

    D   250 mL propranolol 50 mg/5 mL oral solution and 300 mL dipyridamole 50 mg/5 mL solution

    E   320 mL propranolol 50 mg/5 mL oral solution and 300 mL dipyridamole 50 mg/5 mL solution

13 Potassium permanganate solution 1 in 4000 is prepared from a stock of 20 times this strength. How much potassium permanganate will be needed to make sufficient stock solution if a patient uses 100 mL of the diluted solution each day for 5 days?

    A   100 mg
    B   125 mg
    C   250 mg
    D   400 mg
    E   500 mg

14 Given a 5% w/v solution of triclosan, what volume is required to make 250 mL of a 2% w/v solution?

    A   20 mL
    B   40 mL
    C   80 mL
    D   100 mL
    E   140 mL

Directions for Questions 15–18. For each numbered question select the one lettered option that is most closely related to it. Within the group of questions each lettered option may be used once, more than once, or not at all.

Questions **15 and 16** concern the following quantities:

    A   0.09 g
    B   4.05 g
    C   6.3 g
    D   7.55 g
    E   7.87 g

Select, from A to E above, which is the amount of sodium chloride required to make each of these solutions:

15 900 mL of a 100 ppm sodium chloride solution.

16 700 mL of a 5% w/v glucose and 0.9% w/v sodium chloride solution.

Questions **17 and 18** concern the following quantities:

    A   0.21 g
    B   0.22 g
    C   0.875 g
    D   1.068 g
    E   1.55 g

Select, from A to E above, which is appropriate:

17 The weight of calcium in 20 calcium gluconate tablets (calcium gluconate 600 mg tablets – calcium 53.4 mg – Ca^{2+} 1.35 mmol)

18 The weight of sodium fluoride contained in 60 mL En-De-Kay Fluodrops. En-De-Kay Fluodrops: sodium fluoride 550 micrograms (F$^-$ 250 micrograms)/0.15 mL).

Directions for Questions 19 and 20. The questions in this section are followed by three responses. **ONE** or **MORE** of the responses is (are) correct. Decide which of the responses is (are) correct. Then choose:

    A If 1, 2 and 3 are correct
    B If 1 and 2 only are correct
    C If 2 and 3 only are correct
    D If 1 only is correct
    E If 3 only is correct

Directions summarised:

A	B	C	D	E
1, 2, 3	1, 2 only	2, 3 only	1 only	3 only

19 The formula for 100 tablets is:
    Paracetamol 50 g
    Codeine hemihydrate 800 mg
    Caffeine 3 g
    Lactose 20 g
    Which of the following is/are correct?

      1 16 tablets contain 0.128 g codeine hemihydrate
      2 A patient taking two tablets four times daily for 3 days ingests 4.8 g lactose from these tablets
      3 32 tablets contain 960 mg caffeine

20 Which of the following is/are correct?

      1 In order to make 300 g of 2.5% w/w calamine in emulsifying ointment BP, 7.5 g calamine are required
      2 250 mL of a 1.14% w/v solution of povidone–iodine contains 2.85 g of the drug
      3 4 × 250 mg nitrazepam tablets will be required to make 100 mL of a 50 mg/5 mL nitrazepam suspension

PRACTICE TEST 2 – ANSWERS

1 D
Dose is now 5 micrograms before lunch and 10 micrograms before his evening meal, so each day the patient is going to use 15 micrograms
Stock of 2 × 5 microgram/dose, prefilled, 60-dose pens, so between the two pens has 120 × 5 microgram doses
In a day going to use 15 micrograms = 3 × 5 microgram doses
Number of days = total doses available/number of doses used per day
= 120 × 5 micrograms doses/3 × 5 micrograms doses
= 40 days.
Therefore, the correct answer is D.

2 A
Final solution has a strength of 0.005% = 0.005 g potassium permanganate/100 mL
Patient to do a 1 in 10 dilution to produce solution of 0.005% strength
Strength of solution dispensed to patient = 0.05%
0.05% means 0.05 g potassium permanganate/100 mL solution
Need to prepare 2 L of 0.05% solution, so need to calculate the amount of potassium permanganate in this 2 L
0.05% = 0.05 g per 100 mL = 0.05 × 20 g per 2000 mL = 1 g = 1000 mg
Now need to work how out many 400 mg tablets to be used to give 1 g
Number of tablets = 1000/400 = 2.5 tablets.
Therefore, the correct answer is A.

3 D
Morphine sulphate 40 mg every 4 hours – 40 mg × 6/24 hours = 240 mg daily
Therefore the correct answer is D.

4 C
1200 mg in 4 L = 1200 mg/4000 mL
To get percentage strength need to calculate the amount in grams potassium permanganate in 100 mL water
1200/40 mg/100 mL = 30 mg/100 mL = 0.03 g in 100 mL = 0.03%.
Therefore, the correct answer is C.

5 D
Dose: 2.5 mg/kg every 8 h
Patient's weight: 30 kg, so dose is 2.5×30 mg every 8 h = 75 mg every 8 h
Injection strength is 40 mg/mL = 1 mg/(1/40) mL
75 mg in 75/40 mL = 1.875 mL.
Therefore, the correct answer is D.

6 A
7.5 mg/kg twice daily for 20-kg child equates with $(7.5 \times 20 \times 2)$ mg daily
= 300 mg daily
Epilim liquid is 200 mg/5 mL, so need $(300/200) \times 5$ mL daily = 7.5 mL daily
November has 30 days, so in November will use 30×7.5 mL = 225 mL.
Therefore, the correct answer is A.

7 B
Dose: 2 mg/m^2 daily in two doses, so single dose of 1 mg/m^2
For this patient this equates with 1×0.42 mg = 0.42 mg = 420 micrograms
Drug E syrup concentration is 500 micrograms/mL
= 1 microgram/(1/500) mL
420 micrograms in 420/500 mL = 0.84 mL.
Therefore, the correct answer is B.

8 D
$k_{el} = 0.693/t_{1/2}$
so $k_{el} \times t_{1/2} = 0.693$
and $0.924 \text{ h}^{-1} \times t_{1/2} = 0.693$
$t_{1/2} \text{(h)} = 0.693/0.924 = 0.75$ h = 0.75×60 min = 45 min
Therefore the serum concentration will reduce by 50% every 45 min
9am–12pm is a time interval of 3 h = 180 min
Number of half-lives occurring from 9 am to 12 pm = 180/45 = 4
Serum concentration will reduce as follows:
$50 \rightarrow 25 \rightarrow 12.5 \rightarrow 6.25 \rightarrow 3.125$ mg/L
3.125 mg/L = 3.125 micrograms/mL.
Therefore, the correct answer is D.

9 E
$$Cl_{Cr} = \frac{98 - 0.8 \times (\text{patient's age in years} - 20)}{\text{serum creatinine (mg/dL)}}$$
$Cl_{Cr} = 98 - 0.8 \times (45 - 20)/3$
$Cl_{Cr} = 26$ mL/min per 1.73 m^2

$Cl_{Cr} = (26/1.73)$ mL/min per m^2
$Cl_{Cr} = (26/1.73 \times 1.8)$ mL/min for Brian
$Cl_{Cr} \approx 27.05$ mL/min.
Therefore, the correct answer is E.

10 B
If the solution is 1 in 5000, there is 1.0 g in 5000 mL solution
In 500 mL, there is $(1/5000) \times 500 = 0.1$ g = 100 mg
In 100 mL, there is $(1/5000) \times 100 = 0.02$ g = 20 mg
In 1000 mL, there is $(1/5000) \times 1000 = 0.2$ g = 200 mg
In 300 mL, there is $(1/5000) \times 300 = 0.06$ g = 60 mg.
Therefore, the correct answer is B.

11 D
Working backwards from the final solution, we have 0.2% w/v, which equates to 0.2 g chlorhexidine gluconate in 100 mL solution
Multiplying by 30 gives the concentration of the original stock solution, which is, therefore, 6% w/v
This equates with 6 g in 100 mL
As we are starting with 20 mL stock solution, we need $20/100 \times 6$ g, which is equal to 1.2 g chlorhexidine gluconate.
Therefore, the correct answer is D.

12 E
Dipyridamole 300 mg daily in three divided doses $\rightarrow 300 \times 10$ mg over 10 days = 3000 mg
Dipyridamole 50 mg/5 mL solution = 1 mg/0.1 mL or 3000 mg in 300 mL
Propranolol 320 mg daily $\rightarrow 320 \times 10$ mg over 10 days = 3200 mg
Propranolol 50 mg/5 mL oral solution = 1 mg/0.1 mL
3200 mg in 320 mL.
Therefore, the correct answer is E.

13 B
1 in 4000 diluted solution = 1 g in 4000 mL diluted solution
Over the 5 days will use 100 mL $\times 5 = 500$ mL
This 500 mL will contain $1/4000 \times 500$ g = 0.125 g = 125 mg
The volume of stock solution is immaterial because still need it to contain the same weight of potassium permanganate.
Therefore, the correct answer is B.

14 D
2% w/v solution contains 2 g in 100 mL, or 2 × 2.5 g in 250 mL = 5 g
5% w/v solution contains 5 g in 100 mL, or 1 g in 20 mL
Therefore, 5 g found in 100 mL, which is the volume required to make the diluted solution.
Therefore, the correct answer is D.

15 A
100 ppm = 100 g in 1000 000 mL solution
= 100/1000 000 g in 1 mL solution = 1/10 000 g in 1 mL
= 100 × 900/1000 000 g in 900 mL = 0.09 g.
Therefore, the correct answer is A.

16 C
0.9% w/v = 0.9 g in 100 mL
= 0.9 × 7 g in 700 mL = 6.3 g.
Therefore, the correct answer is C.

17 D
Each calcium gluconate tablet contains 53.4 mg calcium
Therefore 53.4 mg × 20 mg calcium in 20 tablets = 1068 mg
= 1.068 g.
Therefore, the correct answer is D.

18 B
Sodium fluoride 550 micrograms/0.15 mL
So in 1 mL there is 550/0.15 micrograms
In 60 mL there are 550 × 60/0.15 micrograms
= 220 000 micrograms
= 220 mg = 0.22 g
Therefore, the correct answer is B.

19 A
1   If 800 mg codeine hemihydrate is required for 100 tablets, each tablet must contain 8 mg
      Accordingly, 16 tablets contain 128 mg codeine hemihydrate = 0.128 g.
2   The patient takes 8 tablets/day for 3 days = 24 tablets
      100 tablets contain 20 g lactose
      (20/100) × 24 = 4.8 g lactose.

3   If 3 g caffeine are required for 100 tablets, each tablet must contain 30 mg
    $32 \times 30 = 960$ mg caffeine.
    All three statements are true.
Therefore, the correct answer is A.

20 A
1   2.5% of 300 g = 7.5 g of calamine required.
2   1.14% w/v = 1.14 g povidone–iodine/100 mL
    Therefore, 1.14×2.5 g in 250 mL = 2.85 g.
3   Nitrazepam 50 mg/5 mL suspension
    1 mL contains 50/5 mg, so 100 mL contains $100 \times (50/5)$ mg = 1000 mg
    Each nitrazepam tablet = 250 mg, so 1000/250 tablets required = 4.
All three statements are true, therefore the correct answer is A.

PRACTICE TEST 3 QUESTIONS

Directions for Questions 1–14. Each of the questions or incomplete statements in this section is followed by five suggested answers. Select the best answer in each case.

1   Sodium nitroprusside is being prescribed for a 75-kg patient in hypertensive crisis; 50 mg sodium nitroprusside has been diluted to 1000 mL in a 5% glucose infusion. The drug is to be administered to the patient at an initial rate of 0.5 microgram/kg per min and then increased in steps of 500 ng/kg per min at 5-min intervals. Which of the following is the infusion rate 17 min after treatment is commenced?

   A   1 mL/min
   B   1.5 mL/min
   C   2 mL/min
   D   2.5 mL/min
   E   3 mL/min

2   The formula for Potassium Citrate Mixture, BP states that 300 mL double-strength chloroform water is required per 1 L of the final mixture. What volume of concentrated chloroform water is required to prepare 2 L of this mixture if the double-strength chloroform water is made from concentrated chloroform water?

   A   15 mL
   B   20 mL
   C   25 mL
   D   30 mL
   E   35 mL

3   Ferrous gluconate 300 mg tablets are currently unavailable from manufacturers due to a supply issue with one of the inactive ingredients. You regularly dispense this tablet for Miss K at a dose of two twice daily. After a discussion with her prescriber you both agree to substitute her regular tablet with Sytron elixir at a suitable dose that contains approximately equivalent iron content. Which of the following is a suitable dose of Sytron elixir for Miss K?
   Ferrous gluconate 300 mg tablets contain 35 mg iron
   Sytron elixir: sodium feredetate 190 mg equivalent to 27.5 mg iron/ 5 mL

    A   10 mL three times daily
    B   10 mL morning and lunch and 5 mL at night
    C   10 mL morning and night
    D   5 mL three times daily
    E   5 mL at night

4   What weight of fluocinolone acetonide is present in 60 g Synalar gel (fluocinolone acetonide 0.025%)?

    A   0.015 g
    B   0.025 g
    C   0.15 g
    D   0.25 g
    E   1.25 g

5   Mrs F has haemorrhoids and has been prescribed Ultraproct suppositories. She has to use the suppositories at a dose of one twice daily for 5 days, then one every other day for a week. Over the course of the treatment how much fluocortolone caproate will Mrs F have used?
Ultraproct suppository: cinchocaine hydrochloride 1 mg, fluocortolone caproate 630 micrograms, fluocortolone pivalate 610 micrograms

    A   8190 mg
    B   7265 mg
    C   6381 mg
    D   5472 mg
    E   4553 mg

6   Mrs J is prescribed oxygen at a high flow rate of 4 L/min. How many complete days of therapy will she have been dispensed if she is dispensed three size F (1360 L) cylinders of oxygen to use for 6 h/day?

    A   1 day
    B   2 days
    C   3 days
    D   4 days
    E   5 days

7   A ward registrar requires an intravenous (IV) infusion of 500 mL sodium chloride 0.18% and glucose 4% to be administered over 100 min to an elderly patient. The IV giving set being used has a flow rate of 5 drops/mL. Which of the following is a suitable drop rate?

A   20 drops/min
B   25 drops/min
C   200 drops/min
D   200 drops/h
E   250 drops/min

8   George weighs 68 kg and requires drug H at a dose of 3 mg/kg per day in four divided doses. Drug H is available as 10 mg capsules. What is the total daily amount of drug H ideally required by George and how many capsules would he take for each dose in practice?

A   204 mg and 15 capsules
B   204 mg and 5 capsules
C   200 mg and 5 capsules
D   105 mg and 5 capsules
E   105 mg and 10 capsules

9   Which of the following is the elimination rate constant (k_{el}) for drug C, which has an elimination half-life $(t_{1/2})$ of 1.5 h, given that $k_{el} = 0.693/t_{1/2}$? (You may assume that the elimination is described by a first-order process.)

A $0.099\ h^{-1}$
B $0.462\ h^{-1}$
C $1.98\ h^{-1}$
D $2.16\ h^{-1}$
E $5.941\ h^{-1}$

10 Elizabeth has been given an emergency 4.5 mg dose of drug F by a doctor after presenting at her local 'out-of-hours' clinic. The elimination half-life of drug F is 0.5 h and it follows first-order kinetics. How much of this drug will remain in her system 2 h after the administration, assuming that complete absorption and distribution have occurred?

A 0.28125×10^{-6} g
B 2.8125×10^{-6} g
C 28.125×10^{-6} g
D 281.25×10^{-6} g
E 2812.5×10^{-6} g

11 Which of the following is the best estimate of the creatinine clearance (Cl_{Cr}) for Hannah, a 66-year-old patient, who weighs 58 kg and has a 140 micromole/L serum creatinine concentration? For females:

$$Cl_{Cr} \text{ (mL/min)} = \frac{1.04 \ (140 - \text{age}) \times \text{weight (kg)}}{\text{serum creatinine (micromoles/L)}}$$

    A   0.36 L/h
    B   1.91 L/h
    C   2.15 L/h
    D   3.48 L/h
    E   3.64 L/h

12 YHR pharmaceuticals produces a batch of compressed tablets every fortnight containing 450 mg active ingredient with a mean tablet weight of 0.9 g. Which of the following is the weight of active ingredient that will be required for a total batch size of 6000 kg?

    A   6000 kg
    B   4000 kg
    C   3000 kg
    D   2500 kg
    E   1800 kg

13 You have in your pharmacy an unopened 30 g tube of Locoid Lipocream (hydrocortisone butyrate 0.1%). Which of the following is the amount of Lipobase cream required for diluting 10 g Locoid Lipocream to a concentration of 0.0025% hydrocortisone butyrate?

    A   250 g
    B   390 g
    C   450 g
    D   575 g
    E   600 g

14 An ointment has the following formula:
Sulphur 4 %w/w
Salicylic acid 10 %w/w
Yellow Soft Paraffin, BP to 100 %w/w
Which of the following are the amounts of sulphur and salicylic acid required to produce 25 g of this ointment?

    A   1 g sulphur and 2.5 g salicylic acid
    B   2.5 g sulphur and 1 g salicylic acid
    C   5 g sulphur and 1 g salicylic acid
    D   8 g sulphur and 8 g salicylic acid
    E   8 g sulphur and 16 g salicylic acid

Directions for Questions 15–18. For each numbered question select the one lettered option that is most closely related to it. Within the group of questions each lettered option may be used once, more than once, or not at all.

Question 15–17 concern the following quantities:

    A   0.21 g
    B   0.63 g
    C   0.87 g
    D   1.08 g
    E   1.5 g

Select, from A to E above, which is appropriate:

15 The total amount of Drug G administered to an adult patient weighing 70.0 kg after 10 days' treatment if he requires a single intravenous daily dose of 0.9 mg/kg body weight of Drug G.

16 The weight of nabumetone in 3 capsules of an experimental analgesic formulation with the following formula for 100 capsules:
Nabumetone   50 g
Codeine phosphate 3 g
Lactose   20 g

17 The weight of sodium fluoride contained in 75 mL Duraphat '2800 ppm' toothpaste (sodium fluoride 0.619%).

Question 18 concerns the following quantities:

    A   0.09 g
    B   4.05 g
    C   6.3 g
    D   7.55 g
    E   7.87 g

Select, from A to E above, which is the amount of sodium chloride required to make this solution.

18 450 mL of a 0.9% w/v sodium chloride solution

Directions for Questions 19 and 20. The questions in this section are followed by three responses. ONE or MORE of the responses is (are) correct. Decide which of the responses is (are) correct. Then choose:

A   If 1, 2 and 3 are correct
B   If 1 and 2 only are correct
C   If 2 and 3 only are correct
D   If 1 only is correct
E   If 3 only is correct

Directions summarised:

A	B	C	D	E
1, 2, 3	1, 2 only	2, 3 only	1 only	3 only

19 Diclofenac tablets contain 50 mg diclofenac sodium. (RMM: diclofenac, $C_{14}H_{11}Cl_2NO_2$ = 296.1 g/mol; diclofenac sodium, $C_{14}H_{10}Cl_2NO_2.Na$ = 318.1 g/mol.) Which of the following is/are correct?

    1   28 tablets contain 1.3 g diclofenac
    2   7.5 g diclofenac sodium would be required to prepare 56 tablets
    3   636.2 g diclofenac sodium contains 2 mol sodium ions

20 Mepyramine maleate is released from a hydrogel-based delivery system in a zero-order fashion, such that the amount of drug, x, released after time t is given by $x = kt$, where k is the zero-order rate constant for this release process. Which of the following is/are correct?

    1   If the zero-order rate constant is 8 mmol/h, then 32 mmol mepyramine maleate are released after 6 h
    2   If 60 mmol are released after 14 h, then the zero-order rate constant is 5.60 mmol/h
    3   If the zero-order rate constant is 35 mmol/h, then 280 mmol mepyramine maleate are released after 8 h

PRACTICE TEST 3 – ANSWERS

1 E

Need to define the dose over each 5-min interval:

0–5 min: 0.5 microgram/kg per min

5–10 min: 1 microgram/kg per min (remember 500 ng = 0.5 mg)

10–15 min: 1.5 micrograms/kg per min

15–20 min: 2 micrograms/kg per min

The question asks about the rate of infusion 17 min after treatment is commenced, so only need to work further with the dose 2 micrograms/kg per min

The patient weighs 75 kg, so dose = 2 × 75 micrograms/min

= 150 micrograms/min

The solution being administered has a strength of 50 mg/1000 mL

= 50 000 micrograms/1000 mL

Need to work out the volume of solution that will contain 150 micrograms and this will be the volume to be administered every minute:

50 000 micrograms/1000 mL

5000 micrograms/100 mL

500 micrograms/10 mL

50 micrograms/mL

150 micrograms/3 mL

Therefore, rate from 15 min to 20 min = 3 mL/min.

Therefore, the correct answer is E.

2 D

Potassium Citrate Mixture, BP: double-strength chloroform water 300 mL/1000 mL

Within a 2 L volume Potassium Citrate Mixture, BP will have 600 mL double-strength chloroform water

Double-strength chloroform water has a concentration of 1 in 20

This means that, to prepare 20 mL double-strength chloroform water, need to use 1 mL concentrate

So to prepare 600 mL need 600/20 mL of concentrate

= 30 mL.

Therefore, the correct answer is D.

3 B

Current medication: two ferrous gluconate 300 mg tablets twice daily

= 2 × 35 mg iron twice daily
= 70 mg twice daily = 140 mg daily
So need to calculate an equivalent iron dose in elixir:
Sytron elixir 27.5 mg iron/5 mL, so 5.5 mg in 1 mL
Volume of elixir that will provide 140 mg iron
= 140/5.5 ≈ 25.45 mL
Therefore would change dose to 25 mL/day and appropriate dose from options is 10 mL in the morning and at lunch, and 5 mL at night.
Therefore the correct answer is B.

4 A
Fluocinolone acetonide 0.025%: 0.025 g in 100 g gel
0.025/100 × 60 g in 60 g gel
= 0.015 g.
Therefore, the correct answer is A.

5 A
Days 1–5 one twice daily = total of 10 suppositories
1 week of 7 days @ dose of one every other day = three suppositories
Therefore, total of 13 suppositories used
Each suppository contains 630 mg fluocortolone caproate
Total used = 13 × 630 mg = 8190 mg.
Therefore, the correct answer is A.

6 C
Flow rate = 4 L/min for 6 h/day means that she will use 4 × 60 × 6 L/day
= 1440 L/day
Each cylinder contains 1360 L, so in three dispensed cylinders will have been supplied 4080 L
Number of days oxygen will last = 4080/1360
= 3 days.
Therefore, the correct answer is C.

7 B
500 mL to be given over 100 min = 500 mL/100 min
5 drops per 1 mL, so rate is ([500 × 5] drops/100 min) = 2500/100 drops/min
= 25 drops/min.
Therefore, the correct answer is B.

8 B
Dose: 3 mg/kg per day in four divided doses, so 68×3 mg daily in four divided doses
= 204 mg daily in four divided doses.
Each dose to be 51 mg
$\approx 5 \times 10$ mg capsules.
Therefore, the correct answer is B.

9 D
$k_{el} = 0.693/1.5$ h
= 0.462 h^{-1}.
Therefore, the correct answer is B.

10 D
2 h/0.5 h = 4, so four half-lives have occurred during the 4 h:
4.5 mg $\rightarrow$ 2.25 mg $\rightarrow$ 1.125 mg $\rightarrow$ 0.5625 mg $\rightarrow$ 0.28125 mg
So, after 2 h the amount of drug F left is 0.28125 mg
0.28125 mg = 2.8125×10^{-4} g = 281.25×10^{-6} g.
Therefore, the correct answer is D.

11 B
$$Cl_{cr} \text{ (mL/min)} = \frac{1.04 \, (140 - 66) \times 58 \text{ (kg)}}{140 \text{ (micromoles/L)}}$$
= 31.88 mL/min
Answers given in litres per hour, so need to convert Hannah's clearance to these units
$Cl_{Cr} = 31.88 \times 60$ mL/h = $(31.88 \times 60)/1000$ L/h
=1.91 L/h.
Therefore, the correct answer is B.

12 C
Every 0.9 g tablet contains 450 mg active drug
Therefore, 900/450 means half of each tablet is active ingredient
Accordingly, half of the batch size of 6000 kg must be active ingredient
6000/2 = 3000
Therefore 3000 kg active ingredient required to produce 6000 kg compressed tablets.
Therefore, the correct answer is C.

13 B
Dilution factor = (initial concn)/(final concn) = (0.1%)/(0.0025%) = 40
Therefore, the original cream needs to be diluted 1 in 40, i.e. 1 part Locoid
Lipocream and 39 parts Lipobase cream
Quantity of Lipobase cream required = 39 × 10 g = 390 g.
Therefore, the correct answer is B.

14 A
Sulphur required = 4% of 25 g
= 4/100 × 25 = 1 g
Salicylic acid required = 10% of 25 g = 2.5 g.
The correct answer is A.

15 B
The daily dose required = (0.9 mg/kg) × (70 kg) = 63.0 mg. After 10 days,
he will have received 63.0 mg × 10 = 630.0 mg or 0.63 g.
Therefore, the correct answer is B.

16 E
If 50 g of nabumetone are required for 100 capsules, then each capsule must
contain 0.5 g. Accordingly, 3 capsules must contain 1.50 g of nabumetone.
Therefore, the correct answer is E.

17 A
2800 ppm = 2800 g sodium fluoride per 1000 000 mL toothpaste
2800/1000 000 g per 1 mL
2800 × 100/1000 000 g per 100 mL = 0.28 g/100 mL
(0.28 g × 75 mL)/100 mL = 0.21 g.
Therefore, the correct answer is A.

18 B
0.9% sodium chloride solution = 0.9 g in 100 mL solution
0.9/100 g in 1 mL solution
0.9 × 450/100 g in 450 mL
= 4.05 g.
Therefore, the correct answer is B.

19 D
1   Diclofenac: diclofenac sodium
     296.1:318.1

x:50

Cross-multiplying, we have: 14 805 = (318.1)x

x = 46.54 mg

This is the amount of diclofenac in one tablet

Accordingly, the amount of diclofenac in 28 tablets is 28 × 46.54 mg

= 1303.12 mg

= 1.3 g.

2　There is 50 mg diclofenac sodium in one tablet, so 56 tablets must contain 56 × 50 mg = 2800 mg

= 2.8 g.

3　636.2 g diclofenac sodium is equivalent to 2 mol diclofenac sodium

As diclofenac and sodium are in a molar ratio of 1:1 in diclofenac sodium, 636.2 g diclofenac sodium contains 2 mol sodium ions.

Overall, only statement 1 is true, so the correct answer is D.

20 E

1　$x = kt$

= 8(6)

= 48 mmol.

2　$x = kt$

60 = k(14)

k = 4.29 mmol/h.

3　$x = kt$

= 35(8)

= 280 mmol.

Overall, only 3 is true, so the correct answer is E.

Index

absorbance, 145, 149, 161, 163
absorption, 79, 84, 95, 99
adrenaline, 1, 19, 42, 57
alcohol, 4, 20, 149, 163
Alkaline Gentian, Mixture, BP, 106, 124
allopurinol, 6, 22, 109, 126
aloxiprin, 120, 133
Altacite Plus suspension, 46, 60
aluminium hydroxide, 171, 178
Alupent syrup, 109, 126
5-aminolevulinic acid, 143, 146, 159, 161
  hydrochloride, 5, 17, 21, 30, 104, 123, 142, 155, 159, 168
aminophylline, 76, 93, 144, 160, 170, 177
  dihydrate, 144, 160
Ammonia and Ipecacuanha, BP, 118, 131
ammonium
  bicarbonate, 118, 131
  chloride, 143, 160
amoxicillin, 10, 25, 106, 116, 124, 130, 140, 157
  trihydrate, 140, 157
anise water, 118, 131
Aromatic Magnesium Carbonate Mixture, BP, 170, 177
ascorbic acid, 110, 127
aspirin, 120, 133
atenolol, 3, 20
Ativan, 116, 130

beclometasone, 11, 25
belladonna tincture, 117, 131
bendroflumethiazide, 152, 165

benzocaine, 112, 128
benzodiazepine, 71, 90
betamethasone
  acetate, 144, 160
  dipropionate, 144, 160
  valerate, 106, 114, 124, 129, 144, 160
Betnovate ointment, 114, 129
bioavailability, 67, 73, 74, 75, 76, 77, 78, 79, 80, 84, 85, 86, 87, 91, 92, 93, 94, 95, 96, 99, 100, 101
bismuth subnitrate, 115, 118, 130, 132
body surface area, 14, 28, 36, 48, 53, 62, 183, 189
British National Formulary, 33, 65
Brufen granules, 40, 56
Byetta, 182, 188

caffeine, 120, 133, 187, 191
calamine, 105, 123, 170, 176
  cream, 12, 27
  ointment, 9, 23, 187, 192
Calcijex (calcitriol), 49, 63
calcium
  carbonate, 4, 21
  chloride hexahydrate, 143, 159
  gluconate, 186, 191, 197, 202
camphor water, 118, 131
capsules, 34, 37, 48, 50, 52, 54, 62, 64, 107, 119, 125, 132, 140, 141, 157, 158, 195, 201
captopril, 117, 131
carbamazepine, 11, 25, 84, 99
carbocysteine, 109, 126
CellCept suspension, 34, 52, 172, 178

Celsius, degrees, 153, 166
Cetomacrogol Cream, BP, 12, 26
chemistry, 137
  answers, 156–68
  questions, 138–55
child dosage regimes, 3, 11, 20, 25,
    35, 36, 38, 40, 43, 44, 45, 47, 48,
    49, 50, 51, 53, 54, 56, 58, 59, 60,
    62, 63, 64, 80, 95, 169, 170, 176,
    177, 183, 189
  with renal function impairment, 43,
    58
Chloral Elixir, Paediatric, BP, 108, 125
chloral hydrate, 108, 125
chlorhexidine gluconate, 5, 14, 16, 21,
    27, 30, 107, 125, 184, 190
chloroform water, 173, 179
  concentrated, 193, 199
  double-strength, 16, 30, 107, 110,
    114, 118, 124, 127, 129, 131,
    193, 199
cimetidine, 8, 23
cinchocaine hydrochloride, 194, 200
clearance, 72, 84, 91, 100
clobetasone butyrate, 108, 125
clotrimazole, 115, 120, 130, 133
coal tar, 110, 127
codeine
  hemihydrate, 154, 167, 187, 191
  hydrochloride, 116, 131
  linctus, 4, 20
  phosphate, 107, 125, 154, 167
  sesquihydrate, 154, 167
Codeine Linctus, BP, 119, 132
Codeine Linctus, Paediatric, BP, 119,
    132
copper sulphate, 3, 19, 184, 190
cortisone, 141, 158
  acetate, 141, 158
creams, 12, 26, 27, 106, 120, 121,
    124, 133, 134
  dilution, 104, 108, 117, 123, 125,
    131, 196, 202
creatinine clearance, 43, 58, 67, 69,
    70, 71, 72, 76, 77, 78, 79, 85, 87,
    88, 89, 90, 91, 93, 94, 95, 101,
    184, 189, 195, 201
cyclophosphamide, 109, 126

Daktacort cream, 153, 166

danaparoid sodium, 40, 56
degradation reactions, 142, 143, 147,
    148, 152, 158, 159, 162, 163, 166
desferrioxamine mesilate, 46, 60
dexamethasone, 14, 28, 171, 177
dexamfetamine sulphate, 48, 62
diamorphine hydrochloride, 43, 45,
    58, 60
diclofenac, 140, 157, 198, 203
  sodium, 40, 56, 111, 127, 140, 157,
    198, 203
dicycloverine hydrochloride, 122, 134
digoxin, 67, 74, 76, 77, 78, 80, 85,
    87, 91, 93, 94, 95, 101
dilutions, 1
  answers, 19–31
  questions, 2–18
dimercaprol, 46, 60
dipyridamole, 185, 190
disintegration constant, 150, 151, 164
dispensing, 103
  answers, 123–35
  questions, 104–22
displacement value, 114, 115, 117,
    118, 130, 131, 132, 172, 179
domperidone, 122, 134
dopamine hydrochloride, 42, 57
dopexamine hydrochloride, 39, 55
dorzolamide hydrochloride, 112, 128
dosing, 33
  answers, 52–64
  questions, 34–51
doxorubicin, 110, 126
drinking water, 15, 28
  fertiliser residues, 9, 24
Duraphat '2800 ppm' toothpaste, 197,
    202

ear drops, 113, 122, 129, 135
Ebixa, 41, 57
elderly patients
  creatinine clearance, 195, 201
  dosing, 35, 41, 52, 57
  pharmacokinetics, 66, 67, 68, 70,
    71, 72, 76, 77, 87, 88, 89, 90, 91,
    93
elimination half-life, 66, 70, 71, 72,
    87, 89, 90, 172, 178, 195, 201
elimination rate constant, 66, 70, 71,
    87, 89, 90, 184, 189, 195, 201

En-De-Kay
  Fluodrops, 186, 191, 197, 202
  mouth rinse, 171, 178
enoximone, 47, 61
Epanutin, 35, 53
Epilim, 183, 189
epoietin beta, 50, 63
ergometrine maleate, 116, 131
erythromycin, 6, 22, 141, 158
  ethyl succinate, 111, 127
  lactobionate, 141, 158
Erythroped suspension, 6, 22
esterase, 155, 168
estradiol, 119, 132
estriol, 119, 132
ethambutol, 14, 27
ethanol, 10, 25
ethylenediamine, 144, 160
etoposide, 48, 62
Eumovate, 108, 125
exenatide, 182, 188
eye drops, 112, 128

Fahrenheit, degrees, 153, 166, 167
ferrous fumarate, 141, 158
ferrous gluconate, 138, 139, 156, 157,
    193, 199
ferrous sulphate, 110, 127
fertiliser residues, 9, 24
first-order kinetics, 66, 68, 70, 71, 75,
    82, 83, 87, 88, 89, 90, 93, 97, 98,
    154, 155, 167, 172, 178, 184,
    189, 195, 201
  decomposition reactions, 142, 147,
    148, 158, 162, 163
  rate constant, 142, 148, 154, 155,
    158, 163, 167
fluconazole, 43, 58
fluocinolone acetonide, 194, 200
fluocortolone
  caproate, 194, 200
  pivalate, 194, 200
fluorescein sodium, 17, 30
fluoride supplements, 15, 28
fluoxetine hydrochloride, 149, 164,
    172, 179
formulae, 1
  answers, 19–31
  questions, 2–18

formulation, 103
  answers, 123–35
  questions, 104–22
fosphenytoin sodium, 37, 54
fucidin suspension, 35, 53
furosemide, 112, 128
fusidic acid, 35, 53
Fybogel Mebeverine, 47, 61

Galenphol paediatric linctus, 175, 180
Galfer
  capsules, 141, 158
  syrup, 139, 157
ganciclovir, 43, 58
Gaviscon Advance, 47, 61
gels, 111, 116, 127, 130
gentamicin, 74, 77, 92, 93, 183, 189
glucose, 6, 21, 112, 128, 186, 191
  injection, 18, 31
  intravenous infusion, 7, 22, 37, 41,
    54, 57, 193, 194, 199, 200
glycerol, 113, 116, 129, 130
glyceryl trinitrate, 105, 123
granules, 138, 156

half-life, 66, 68, 70, 75, 82, 83, 87,
    88, 89, 93, 97, 98, 142, 147, 148,
    154, 158, 162, 163, 167
  radioisotopes, 150, 164
haloperidol, 10, 25, 35, 52
hexylaminolevulinate, 121, 134, 146,
    155, 161, 162, 168
high-performance liquid
    chromatography, 145, 146, 161
hydrocortisone, 117, 131
  butyrate, 196, 202
  cream, 11, 12, 26, 27
  sodium succinate, 107, 125
hydrogen peroxide, 122, 135
Hydrous Ointment, BP, 7, 22
hydroxycarbamide, 50, 64

[131]I, 150, 151, 164
ibuprofen, 40, 56
imiquimod, 151, 165
inhaled salbutamol, 15, 28
injection solution, 6, 22
intramuscular injection, 37, 45, 54, 60

intravenous administration, 35, 53, 172, 174, 178, 180
  bolus, 71, 83, 91, 98
  infusion, 16, 29, 35, 37, 44, 53, 54, 59, 66, 70, 87, 89, 139, 156, 175, 181
    flow rate, 7, 13, 22, 27, 36, 39, 41, 42, 43, 47, 48, 49, 50, 54, 55, 57, 58, 61, 62, 63, 64, 193, 194, 199, 200
    loading dose, 66, 70, 76, 87, 89, 93
  injection, 40, 56, 86, 101
ipecacuanha, 118, 131
iron, 39, 56, 138, 139, 141, 156, 157, 158, 193, 199

Jelliffe equation, 71, 90, 184, 189

Keltrol suspension, 117, 131
ketoconazole, 121, 134
Kolanticon, 122, 134

lactose, 107, 111, 125, 127, 187, 191
Lanoxin, 80, 95
levetiracetam, 67, 69, 87, 88
levothyroxine, 171, 177
lidocaine hydrochloride, 42, 57
light magnesium carbonate, 114, 129
Lipobase cream, 196, 202
liquid medicines, 1, 4, 7, 15, 19, 20, 22, 29, 173, 179
liquorice, 118, 131
lithium, 142, 159
  carbonate, 142, 159
loading dose, 66, 67, 70, 74, 77, 78, 87, 89, 91, 94
lorazepam, 116, 130
Lucoid Lipocream, 196, 202
lymecycline, 140, 157

magnesium
  hydroxide, 34, 52, 171, 178
  trisilicate, 114, 129
Magnesium Trisilicate Mixture, BP, 114, 129
maintenance dose, 73, 74, 79, 85, 91, 92, 94, 100, 101
mefenamic acid, 174, 179

memantine hydrochloride, 41, 57
meptazinol hydrochloride, 37, 54
mepyramine maleate, 198, 203
methanol, 155, 168
methotrexate, 48, 62, 169, 176
methylaminolevulinate, 12, 26, 104, 123, 151, 165
methylcellulose, 116, 130
methylene blue, 17, 30, 111, 127
methylparaben, 116, 130
methylprednisolone sodium succinate, 172, 179
Metvix, 104, 123
Michaelis–Menton model, 73, 91
milrinone lactate, 48, 61
misoprostol, 111, 127
molar absorptivity, 145, 161
moles, 142, 143, 159, 160
Molipaxin, 105, 124
morphine
  hydrochloride, 173, 179
  sulphate, 169, 176, 182, 188
    modified-release capsules, 182, 188
Motilium, 122, 134
mouthwash, 8, 23, 171, 178
Mucodyne, 109, 126
Mucogel, 34, 52, 171, 178
mycophenolate mofetil, 34, 52, 172, 178

Niferex elixir, 39, 56
nitrazepam, 7, 22, 187, 192
Nizoral cream, 121, 134

ointments, 105, 110, 112, 114, 123, 127, 128, 129, 170, 176, 196, 202
opioid analgesia, 45, 60
oral drops, 41, 57
Oramorph oral solution, 169, 176
orciprenaline sulphate, 109, 126
oxycodone hydrochloride, 45, 60
oxygen, 194, 200

paediatric codeine linctus, 4, 20
Paediatric Ferrous Sulphate Mixture, 110, 127
Pamergan-P100, 41, 56
paracetamol, 107, 118, 125, 132, 187, 191

patches, 104, 121, 123, 134
pathlength of spectrometer cell, 145, 161
peak area ratio, 145, 146, 161
peak serum concentration, 77, 93, 184, 189
peppermint emulsion, concentrated, 114, 129
peppermint water, 4, 20
Peptac suspension, 11, 25
pericyazine syrup, 44, 59
pessaries, 115
pethidine hydrochloride, 41, 56
pharmacokinetics, 65
  answers, 87–101
  questions, 66–86
phenindione, 8, 23
phenol, 146, 161
phenoxymethylpenicillin, 113, 129
phenytoin, 5, 21, 35, 53, 73, 84, 91, 100
  sodium, 119, 132
Pholcodine Linctus, BP, 175, 180
Pholcodine Linctus, Strong, BP, 175, 180
phytomenadione, 14, 27
plasma concentration, 72, 73, 76, 78, 79, 81, 82, 83, 84, 90, 91, 93, 94, 96, 97, 98, 99, 100, 172, 174, 178, 180
Plesmet syrup, 138, 156
porfimer sodium, 14, 27, 106, 124
potassium, 47, 61, 143, 160
  chloride, 44, 59, 143, 160, 175, 181
  citrate mixture, 16, 30, 193, 199
  permanganate, 1, 5, 9, 17, 19, 21, 25, 31, 182, 183, 185, 188, 190
povidone–iodine, 187, 192
powder
  for injection, 107, 125
  for oral use, 120, 133
practice tests
  answers, 176–81, 188–92, 199–203
  questions, 169–75, 182–7, 193–8
prednisolone, 7, 11, 22, 26
pro-epanutin, 37, 54
proflavine hemisulphate, 7, 22
promethazine hydrochloride, 41, 56
propranolol, 185, 190
purity, 150, 151, 164, 165

pyrazine 2,5-dipropionic acid, 143, 159

radioactivity, 150, 151, 164, 165
radioisotopes, 150, 151, 164, 165
ranitidine, 3, 20, 80, 96, 139, 156
  hydrochloride, 47, 61, 122, 134, 139, 156
relative molecular mass, 138, 140, 141, 142, 143, 144, 154, 156, 157, 158, 159, 160, 167, 198, 203
renal function, 43, 58, 67, 69, 76, 87, 88, 93
riamactane, 34, 52
rifampicin, 34, 52

salbutamol, 15, 28
  sulphate, 146, 162
salicylic acid, 7, 22, 105, 114, 124, 129, 196, 202
  cream, 11, 25
  lotion, 11, 25
saline infusion, 36, 50, 54, 64
salt factor, 67, 73, 74, 75, 76, 77, 78, 79, 84, 85, 86, 91, 93, 94, 99, 100, 101
saturated aqueous solution, 108, 126
shelf-life, 148, 154, 155, 163, 167
simeticone, 46, 47, 60
sodium, 11, 25, 40, 47, 56, 61, 139, 156
  bicarbonate, 107, 108, 113, 114, 124, 126, 129, 170, 175, 177, 181
  chloride, 6, 21, 138, 139, 140, 156, 157, 175, 181, 186, 191
  intravenous infusion, 16, 29, 42, 58, 120, 133, 194, 200
  solution, 16, 29, 197, 202
  feredetate, 193, 199
  fluoride, 171, 178, 186, 191, 197, 202
  nitroprusside, 49, 62, 193, 199
  valproate, 110, 126, 183, 189
Sodium Chloride Solution, BP, 16, 29
Solaraze gel, 40, 56
solubility, 113, 128
Solvazinc effervescent tablets, 51, 64
spironolactone, 8, 22, 115, 130
starch, 105, 119, 124, 132

stock solutions, 5, 8, 13, 14, 16, 21, 23, 27, 30, 184, 190
storage conditions, 153, 166
subcutaneous infusion, 45, 60
subcutaneous injection, 45, 60
sulfathiazole sodium sesquihydrate, 148, 163
sulphur, 196, 202
    cream, 11, 26
suppositories, 114, 115, 118, 130, 132, 194, 200
suppository base, 114, 115, 117, 130, 131
suspensions, 9, 12, 23, 26, 38, 39, 55, 106, 109, 115, 117, 119, 120, 124, 126, 130, 131, 132, 133
Synalar gel, 194, 200
Syrup, BP, 13, 27
syrups, 86, 101, 108, 109, 125, 126, 183, 189
Sytron elixir, 193, 199

tablets, 6, 7, 8, 11, 14, 17, 22, 23, 26, 28, 31, 41, 44, 48, 57, 59, 62, 86, 101, 109, 111, 112, 126, 127, 128, 182, 188, 193, 199
    weight of active ingredient, 104, 123, 138, 139, 140, 141, 144, 156, 157, 158, 160, 196, 197, 198, 201, 202, 203
target concentration, 74, 76, 91, 93
Tegretol, 11, 25, 84, 99
temperature, 153, 166
Tenormin, 3, 20
terbutaline sulphate, 44, 59
Tetralysal, 140, 157
theophylline, 75, 79, 93, 94, 144, 152, 160, 165
therapeutic index, 73, 91
thermometer readings, 153, 166

Timentin, 78, 94
timolol maleate, 112, 128
toluidine blue O, 121, 134, 155, 168
topiramate, 45, 59
trazodone hydrochloride, 105, 124
triamterene, 150, 164
triclosan, 185, 191
trimethoprim, 8, 23

Ultraproct, 194, 200
units, 1
uracil, 146, 161

valaciclovir, 68, 88
vancomycin hydrochloride, 36, 53
venlafaxine, 76, 93
volume of distribution, 66, 67, 70, 71, 72, 74, 76, 77, 78, 79, 81, 83, 87, 89, 90, 91, 93, 94, 96, 99, 174, 180

Water for Injections, BP, 16, 29, 107, 109, 110, 116, 125, 126, 130, 172, 179
white soft paraffin, 105, 114, 129
White Soft Paraffin, BP, 105, 123, 124

yellow soft paraffin, 110, 127
Yellow Soft Paraffin, BP, 196, 202

Zantac, 3, 20, 122, 134
zero-order kinetics, 152, 165, 198, 203
    decomposition reactions, 142, 147, 159, 162
    rate constant, 142, 147, 152, 159, 162, 165, 198, 203
zinc
    oxide, 1, 19, 105, 110, 123, 124, 127
    sulphate monohydrate, 51, 64